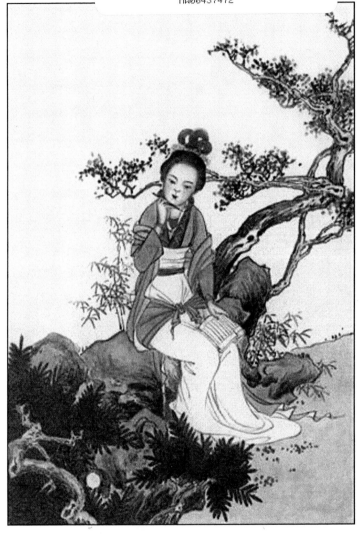

# Feed Your Body, Energize Your Life!

# Feed Your Body, Energize Your Life!

## Dr. Jane Hendricks

❧

### Community of Higher Living Press

*www.communityofhigherliving.com*

Phoenix, Arizona

Community of Higher Living Press
Phoenix, Arizona
*www.communityofhigherliving.com*

Library of Congress Cataloging-in-Publication Data
Hendricks, Jane
    Feed Your Body, Energize Your Life!
Library of Congress Catalog Card Number 2007903322
ISBN 978-0-9795008-0-0

Cover and book design by Tony Stubbs, *www.tjpublish.com*
Photography by Noah Leaf Mendelson, *www.leafgallery.com*

### Disclaimer
All information in this book is provided by Dr. Jane Hendricks for informational purposes only and is not medical advice or diagno-sis, nor is it to be construed as medical advice, medical information, medical diagnosis, or medical prescription for curing, removing, or preventing any disease, or related symptoms.

The author and publisher will not be liable under any contract, negligence, or strict liability or other legal or equitable theory for any special, incidental, indirect, or consequential or exemplary damages arising out of or in connection with this publication.

Printed in the United States of America

# Contents

# Dedication

*To all the students of health.*

# Acknowledgments

I am grateful most of all to the source of all intelligence; for all that has been, is, and ever will be.

To Paramahansa Yogananda for his guidance through the written word and beautiful chants.

To Colleen Ceton who showed me how to teach and empower others.

I am grateful to my students for teaching me how to be a better human being.

To Noah, my divine friend, who reminds me of what's really important in this world – the evolution of our souls.

To all who contributed in making this book what it is today. I am especially grateful to Kathleen Malone for her talent in book cover design, and to Jeanie Riley and Carol Adler for their gifts in the English language.

# Introduction

*In a healthy human state, the spirit-like force that enlivens the material organism as dynamis, governs without restriction and keeps all parts of the organism in admirable, harmonious vital operation, as regards both feelings and functions, so that our indwelling, rational spirit can freely avail itself of this living, healthy instrument for the higher purposes of our existence.*

— Samuel Hahnemann

I am a doctor, not a writer. However I want to share my vision with all those people, like myself, who have decided to take charge of their health. I was licensed as a naturopathic physician in 2003. Naturopathic physicians graduate from four-year graduate medical schools. There are three schools in the nation. In my state, naturopaths can diagnose and treat disease as primary care physicians as well as prescribe pharmaceuticals. The natural modalities that a naturopath is trained in are chiropractic, acupuncture, intravenous therapy, nutrition, medicinal herbs, and homeopathy.

As for nutrition, a typical naturopath will prescribe pharmaceutical grade supplements or intravenous vitamins to a patient. There was very little education on food; instead we learned how to use isolated vitamin supplements to treat disease.

Throughout school and into my first year of practice, I experimented with many different health products for my own health issues and for those of my patients. I had always suffered with digestive problems, mainly constipation and abdominal bloating. I had chronic fatigue and slept 10 to 12 hours per day. I also had hypoglycemia (low blood sugar). I had never eaten a lot of meat before going to medical school. However, I was taught by my instructors to eat meat three times a day to balance my blood sugar and to rid myself of the fungus, *Candida Albicans*.

By the time I graduated, I was the sickest I'd ever been. The stress during the board exams had caused me to have colitis. After I completed my board exams, my intestines shut down and the candida, which caused the abdominal bloating and fatigue, worsened. The fatigue was affecting my quality of life; I was exhausted and dizzy all of the time. I opened up my practice and prescribed to my patients the same things I was doing, because that is all I knew.

Eight months later, a friend introduced me to some Chinese herbal foods. I was reluctant; however, he had the energy I wanted. I decided to try the herbs myself, and I will always be glad and grateful that I did! I have more energy in my mid-thirties than I did as a teenager. For the first time in decades, my abdomen is not distended. My adult acne is gone, my cravings have changed, and my enormous appetite has diminished.

What I will be talking about later is that we eat way too much food because we're starving at a cellular level. So we eat and eat. Just because you have food in your digestive tract doesn't mean you're nourished. If you cannot digest, absorb, and assimilate your food properly, the nutrients are not getting into your cells. Consequently, the undernourished cells continue to send messages of hunger to the brain. Furthermore, if the food you eat is depleted of nutrients or dead, then you are starving. As a result of feeding my body these powerful herbal foods, my body cleansed itself. The bad stuff moved out and my body rebuilt itself. I look at myself today and can't believe it's me.

As I was sharing these foods with my patients, I discovered that I no longer needed to treat disease and symptoms. Diagnosing disease implies that there are different treatments for separate diseases. I watched one patient with Crohn's disease and another with asthma both get well from eating the same foods. A patient suffering from multiple organ imbalances would find resolution of all her myriad symptoms. Rather than treating her individual symptoms, I gave her foods that nourished and cleansed the body.

What really excited me is that as a result of eating these herbal foods, the patients changed their lifestyles, discontinued their stimulants and started exercising on a regular basis. A balanced and cleansed body knows what it wants and doesn't need. Before I learned about these herbal foods, the only patients who got well were those who changed their lifestyles—a total of two people during that first year of practice! The patients who took all the vitamins but never changed their lifestyle were dealing with the same health challenges as when they first came to see me.

A year after beginning the herbal food program, I closed my practice and started teaching classes. I discovered through experience that for the patient to be successful, they needed to learn how the body works and also have a vision of health. I teach the necessity of good food for optimal health and the way the mind impacts every area of our life.

In his book, *Illusions*, Richard Bach tells us: "Within each one of us lies the power of our consent to health and to sickness, to riches and to poverty, to freedom and to slavery; it is we who control these and not another." Your health is already yours. All you have to do is receive the gifts bestowed upon you by the heavens. We are inclined to look outward for our health, as this seems easiest to do. The answers you search for are inside, waiting for your mind to be silent and listen. Fear and worry keep us where we're at. Courage propels us forward. The key is to find your peace, and when you do, all the answers you seek come gushing into your consciousness. The American goal is to capture the gold; the Chinese goal is to capture inner peace.

How did it come to be that 70% of Americans over the age of 40 are suffering from one or more chronic degenerative diseases? Why is it that 62% of Americans are overweight? We grew up relying on commercialized institutions to tell us what to eat. For the past 70 years, our scholastic nutritional education has been paid for by the American Dairy Association, the American Farming Association and the meat industry. McDonald's restaurants should be added to that list, since kids are more familiar with the McDonald's song than the Pledge of Allegiance. The average U.S. child sees 5,000 ads on soda and junk food each week and fast food companies are strategically placed in the public schools. The purpose is clear: to addict the kids so they'll keep buying.

With all of the hospitals and doctors, why aren't the sick getting well? We trust medical doctors to understand why we have certain symptoms and how to bring the body back to health, just as we trust mechanics to diagnose and fix our cars. With my car, I'm willing to take the chance that a mechanic may not know what's wrong with it because I'm not going to invest time in learning how to fix it myself. However, my body is too important to just hand over its fate to someone else. This body was given to me to take care of. It is my responsibility to know how it works and what it needs.

The body has always known how to heal itself. It has an intelligence that science will never comprehend. One of my mentors, a holistic nutritionist, taught that "the brain, when healthy and nourished, sends positive messages to all the cells. There is a healing energy inherent in that message which compels the body back to health by sending out rhythmic patterns that the cells recognize."

Once you understand how the body works, you will be empowered to take care of yourself. That is the primary purpose of this book.

There are three levels of knowing. The first level is to receive the data without discernment. A medical student is simply a receptacle for the input from her professors. When asked a question, the student knows the answer because she's heard the information before. At this level of knowing you don't have to believe the information is true. This is the way medical students survive through school. There is not enough time to question whether the information is valid; the data must be regurgitated on an exam and then you move on.

The second level of knowing is when you have heard the information before, only this time you believe it to be true. For example, most people believe that unconditional love should be practiced by everyone. Does that mean most people practice this sort of love everyday? No, absolutely not. Many of us strive to love unconditionally more minutes today than yesterday. It's an evolving process that may take a lifetime.

The third level of knowing is when you hear it, believe it to be true, and assimilate the information, thereby putting it into everyday practice. Using the example of unconditional love, this individual forgives everyone for their wrongs, has universal compassion, and holds no negative feelings or thoughts towards any other person, stranger or not. The practices for higher living, such as unconditional love or healthy eating, have been downloaded into her subconscious mind or heart. Until you are at this third level of knowing, the techniques that you want to practice sit idly in your conscious mind.

A teacher once said, "A truly educated person is he who can instantly apply to his best advantage the lessons learned through life. And if it's the right thing to do, why would you wait?" Due to an inner separation, an individual may think one thing, feel another, and do something entirely different. With integration of thoughts and feelings comes true power and endless choices.

Hopefully, the wisdom gained from this book will inspire you to begin practicing goodwill towards the earth, your body, and your spirit.

# Chapter One

# You and Mother Nature

*When human energy remains in harmony with the primal forces of heaven and earth, it flourishes and protects the health of the body.*

—Daniel Reid

Universal laws apply to your outer world and your inner world, which is your body and mind. One of these laws is cause and effect. When you put poison or toxins into your body, whether it is a commercial food or a drug, you will experience a toxic reaction. The symptoms may not be evident at first because the body is good at compensating, but at some point you will indeed begin to experience the effect.

We are also putting poison into the soil and acting inhumanely towards animals that share this planet with us. Like the human body, the earth compensates so we may not feel the immediate effect of our actions. However, Mother Nature will prevail and eventually we will experience the environmental and physical effects of our choices.

The human body depends on the planet for its survival and by exploiting its resources we are depriving ourselves of necessary nutrients. People living in industrialized societies have the poorest health; in contrast, natives who live close to nature have no knowledge of chronic degenerative diseases.

We humans cannot extract and assimilate the inorganic minerals of the earth, yet our bodies must have organic minerals in order to survive. We have been given a middleman that can take inorganic minerals from the soil, mix them with light and water, and produce organic minerals. This is the plant. Through the plant, we are able to receive nourishment from the sun and earth. Other essential nutrients that we need from the plant are vitamins, enzymes, and amino acids. By eating the plant in its original state we partake in the goodness of the earth and the heavens.

In fighting with nature, the human race continues to separate itself from The Source which gives all life. The Chinese saw the human body as a microcosm of nature. According to the ancient Chinese philosophy, we have our own internal climates of spring, summer, late summer, autumn, and winter. The Chinese looked to nature to learn about the internal workings of the physical body and found all of the answers to longevity, inner peace and beauty. Unfortunately no money is to be made when the answer is already there. Science, with all of its insecurities, searches endlessly for what is right in front of them. All we have to do is live in harmony with the earth and we have our health.

According to the Taoist, all human life depends upon three treasures that every human being is born with. These are spirit, essence, and energy. The goal of the Taoist is to do the inner work necessary to preserve these treasures throughout the human life span. The first treasure has two parts: the higher or prenatal spirit and the lower, earth-bound postnatal spirit. The higher spirit is the "original light of consciousness," the all-knowing self that resides in the heart. Also called *Shen*, this deep part of us is directly connected to the powers of the universe. Our higher self speaks through feelings and vibrations throughout the body.

The postnatal spirit, which is closer to the earth and resides in the mind, manifests in thought. This is the ego and sense of self. The ego is dualistic, limited, and analytical. The mind controls the body through the nervous system. Therefore, your thoughts are critical to the health of your cells. You can open up the mind by integrating your thoughts and feelings. With integration one may experience inner peace and joy.

My definition of health is not merely the absence of disease. It is that state of perfect emotional, spiritual, and physical well-being. The results you experience in areas of relationships, prosperity and physical health are the ways in which you can measure your level of integration. In other words, your outer world reflects your inner world.

Essence is the second treasure that we are born with. Also called *Jing*, it is our potential energy as in a battery. The body draws from this potential energy as it requires. *Jing* is stored in what the Chinese refer to as the kidneys and is the inner source of growth and decay. In today's highly competitive, high-stress lifestyle, we deplete our essence so rapidly, by the time we reach a certain age most of us start to rely on drugs to keep us alive; passing on to the next dimension barely conscious. I think this is the biggest catastrophe of modern medicine because it deprives us of the honor and dignity of fully experiencing our death. Not to be conscious during this most important transition is for me the biggest crime we can commit on our souls.

Energy is our third treasure. Called *Qi* (chi) in Chinese, it is like an electrical current coursing through the human body. To regenerate as we age, we need to deposit more energy into our battery than we withdraw. To achieve longevity one must harness his energy and not waste it on the desires of the flesh. Dead foods consume our essence, while live foods can replenish it. Emotional disturbances and internal chaos also deplete the essence. Food chemicals, poisonous air and negative TV reports are examples of environmental influences that deplete our energy. One must choose his lifestyle carefully and not be distracted by the "evil energies."

We are born with one form of *Qi* that originates from the life force that pervades the universe through vibrations. This is referred to as the original or prenatal *Qi*. We can access this energy by tapping into our essence that is stored in the adrenal glands. We also obtain energy from our environment, which is the source of postnatal *Qi*. We receive earthly energy from food, water, and herbs. The body extracts the nutrients it needs and blends them with air from the lungs to form "pure human energy."

*Qi* is responsible for protecting the body, keeping it warm and retaining the fluids. It is the source of energy for transforming substances into body fluids. *Shen*, *Jing*, and *Qi* are the three treasures that if harmonized, create the human life force that expresses through the body and mind.

We must start taking care of our planet if we want to survive. The Native Americans walked lightly on the earth for thousands of years, leaving no residue and giving back what they took. They honored their kill and didn't waste anything. Everywhere on the planet modern man has raped the soil. The animals are tormented by the farming industry, which forces them to live in horrendous conditions, only to be tortured again in the slaughtering process. Genetically altered plants are grown on sterile soil and given chemical enemas. Today's consumer must be made aware of the environmental consequences of our food production. Albert Einstein said the following about human health and the environment: "Nothing will benefit human health and increase the chances for survival of life on earth as much as the evolution to a vegetarian diet." Did you know that U.S. livestock graze on roughly 525 million acres in the U.S.—nearly two acres for each person? Five thousand gallons of water are required to grow one pound of beef, versus 49 gallons of water required to grow one pound of apples.

As much as we'd like to ignore it, the human being is a part of the earth, its plants and animals. Are you aware that the human race ends once the plant kingdom is gone? After all, we eat the animals that eat the plants. Yet plants and animals are innocent pawns of our ravenous appetites. When the human lives in harmony with nature, the mind, body and spirit are rejuvenated. The essence is restored and pure joy resides in the heart.

Mother Nature is a perfectionist, and we certainly can appreciate her beauty. Animals in the wild heal themselves quickly or die. Poor quality of life does not exist in the wild kingdom. If a plant has grown up to be weak, Mother Nature pulls it back into her womb to begin again. The fungus that normally grows along the rootlets of the plant consumes it, thereby returning all the minerals back to the soil. When the modern farmer sees the decaying plant being overtaken by the fungus, he "treats" it with fungicides.

*Mycorrhiza*, a fungus that grows along the rootlets of a living plant, helps that plant to select specific minerals for its use. It also protects the plant from the millions of microbes in the soil. By killing the *mycorrhiza* with fungicides, the plant's immune system is destroyed and the bacteria in the soil are free to attack the plant. In addition, the plant can no longer select the necessary minerals it needs to grow and be strong. The weak plant then develops a bacterial infection and becomes feverish in the same way a human gets feverish from the flu. So what does the commercial farmer do? In treating the "sick" plant, he sprays bactericides to kill the bacteria.

Microbial life in the soil has a vital role; its metabolism produces minerals. Use of bactericides kills all microbial life. When the bacteria that make minerals are gone, the topsoil becomes depleted in nutrients. Any plants that grow from sterile soil are weak, and Mother Nature, a perfectionist, will not have deficient plants growing from her soil. Her only choice now is to send for the big guns to take the weak plant down. These are the insects that eat our plants. In response to the presence of insects on his plants, the farmer fights back by spraying pesticides onto the plant.

Currently we are fighting constant battles with uglier and meaner bugs that keep mutating in order to resist the insecticides. According to the EPA, 1.2 billion pounds of insecticides were sprayed on our food in the year 2000. Up until the 1940s we grew all of our food without the use of synthetic chemicals, and the crop output was equal to or greater than it is now.

Now, let's look at the development of a human being in today's society and see if there are any similarities to the development of today's commercially grown plant. A new-born is welcomed to its earthly life with a vaccine; this is followed by more vaccines and boosters given during its first two years of life. These regular invasions to the young immune system never allow it to learn how to defend the body on its own.

At the first sign of a cold, the child is prescribed an antibiotic to kill the bug, which suppresses the immature immune system. Chronic ear infections and runny noses are common among today's youth. Due to a weak immune system, the child develops asthma, chronic bronchitis or some other "itis" ailment and grows up taking immuno-suppressants and anti-inflammatories, two types of drugs that are commonly prescribed when doctors don't know what else to do. These drugs quiet the body by suppressing symptoms. Taken over time, they weaken the immune system to the point where it has no remaining defenses to fight back. By conforming to the allopathic methods of treatment, the human body is made to be dependent on drugs since its birth.

The plant, which is our only source of nutrients, is being genetically engineered so it will survive the onslaught of poisonous sprays. If a plant is deprived of good food, humans, who get their nourishment from plants, will also be deprived. We have deficient plants and deficient humans growing with undeveloped immune systems, dependant on man's chemicals for survival. No wonder cancer, a disease of immunodeficiency, is the number one cause of death in this country! The use of agrichemicals and the corresponding exponential rise in cancer have occurred only in the last 50-60 years. In addition, one in five people are diagnosed with some type of autoimmune disease, which means the confused immune system has turned inward and is attacking itself.

How about the animals we eat? How healthy are they? Due to the filth that the animals live in, breeders administer powerful antibiotics whose amounts increase annually to combat the many bacteria and viruses that have mutated into becoming resistant to the drugs. The amount of antibiotics given routinely to U.S. livestock is 24.6 million pounds. The amount of antibiotics given to Americans each year to treat disease is 3 million pounds.

We have no excuse for being a sick country. We have more hospitals and doctors per capita and better sanitation than any other nation in the world, yet the average American starts deteriorating at the age of 40 and from then on, it's a downhill path. Even our children are degenerating when they should be growing. Did you know that cancer is the number one cause of death in today's youth? Why aren't there rallies and picket signs protesting this disturbing state of affairs? Perhaps because few people are aware of this statistic and the seriousness of the situation.

We cannot depend on the media for our education, since studies on drugs and commercial foods are paid for by their respective industries. Rather, we need to start doing our own research and educate each other on food and the way its production impacts the environment.

# Chapter Two

# Your Cells

*The flame is never the same yet always the same. The matter that makes up the flame at any given instant has vanished by the next instant and has been replaced by fresh matter. What persists in this luminous heart of chemical activity is not the substance but the form. And life itself persists in an analogous, although far more complex, fashion.*

—John Pfeiffer, Life Science Library

In every second that passes, some 50 million cells die and 50 million baby cells are born. You are not the same person you were a minute ago. The body is dynamic and can be divided into infinitely minute particles. The cell itself is made up of much smaller units.

Robert Hook, an English Scientist, came up with the word "cell" in 1663. In 1838, Matthias Schleiden, a German botanist, announced that the cell was the basic structural unit of all vegetable matter. A year later one of his colleagues, Theodor Schwann, stated that "cells are organisms, and entire animals and plants are aggregates of these organisms arranged according to definite laws."

Your cells are your life force. They reflect how you feel about yourself. The human cell can be compared to a metropolis bustling with activity. In a healthy body, no cell is on welfare. Even in starvation and dehydration, the cell works to its best ability in order to perform its functions. The cells are the children of the mind. They have feelings, and need food and water to nourish and cleanse themselves.

All life on earth—whether it is a cluster of bacteria or a great scientist—exists because of photosynthesis and respiration. Through the chemical process of photosynthesis, the plant cell traps a tiny amount of the sun's energy and uses it to convert water from the soil and carbon dioxide from the air into sugar and oxygen. Through respiration, animal cells take in oxygen and use it to turn food into energy. The animal must get glucose, its main fuel, from a plant. It is the plant that takes the "radiant energy" of the sun and transforms it into glucose and oxygen.

Antoinne Bechamp, a medical professor from France in the 1800s, stated that every living thing down to a cell is made up of smaller bodies, which he referred to as microzymes. If the environment in which these bodies live becomes morbid, the microzymes divide and become bacteria; so the birth of bacteria is from within, not without. Henry Lindlahr, M.D., said "the microzyme is a microcosm, the cell its macrocosm, just as man is the macrocosm of the cell, and as the sidereal universe is the macrocosm of man. As the well-being of man depends upon normal nutrition and wholesome surroundings, so also the health of the cell depends upon proper nutrition and drainage. Thus, provided with its essential life requirements, the primary unit of life will develop into the normal cells of the vegetable, animal or human body, not into disease germs or parasites."

These minute living bodies are in the business of feeding, and this has fermentative effects within the body. According to Bechamp, fermentation exists in all living bodies and does not depend on the existence of harmful bacteria. Bechamp's view of the living body is not conducive to the germ theory that says you "catch" bacteria from the outside and get sick. We will talk more about the germ theory in a later chapter.

The modern western view of the cell also recognizes minute bodies that live within every living cell. These are called organelles because they resemble organs. They eat, breathe and move just like the cell in which they live. In fact, it is believed that the mitochondrion, known as the "powerhouse" of the cell, is the descendent of bacteria from early evolutionary history.

Every cell has a membrane around it. The cell membrane, also called the plasma membrane, is a "fluid lipid bilayer," essentially made up of cholesterol and phospholipids. It is through this membrane that the cell eats, drinks and eliminates its wastes. If the human has been eating hard fats, this lipid bilayer becomes stiff rather than supple. Like the intestines of your digestive system, if the cell membrane is dry and stiff, the cell cannot assimilate its nutrients or eliminate wastes. Since every organ of the body is made up of individual cells and the intestines are organs, then it would be logical to conclude that the health of the individual cells of the intestines determines how well a person can absorb their nutrients and eliminate waste.

Across every cell membrane lies an energy potential. This potential depends on the separation of positive and negative charges outside and inside the cell. The resting membrane potential is -70 millivolts. Sodium and potassium, two trace minerals, play a critical role in maintaining this potential. Since the body is composed of 75 to 100 trillion cells, we have considerable energy potential. No one can say they are tired after hearing these numbers. The energy potential of the body can be compared to the energy potential of a battery. The battery is fueled by electricity, whereas the body is fueled by water and enzymes. The Chinese refer to this potential as "essence."

The type, quantity and time of day that we eat determine how much essence we have. Raw plants are energetic foods and give up their essence to the cells of the body. However, when you eat lifeless food, the energy potential of your body is being depleted with every meal due to the enormous energy it takes to break down the dead bodies and make them usable.

For food the cell depends mainly on glucose, although there are exceptions to the rule such as with the cardiac cells. The cell drinks water, which is crucial for all of its processes. The cell also needs oxygen, so it inspires oxygen and expires carbon dioxide. The mitochondrion, which is the energy factory of the cell, takes the glucose and using water and oxygen, converts the glucose into fuel, called ATP. ATP is to a cell what electricity is to a city.

The cell lives in a community with other cells and for its survival must be able to communicate with its countrymen. Cells do not touch each other; rather they are suspended in a gel-like matrix through which messenger chemicals move. Tissue is made up of cells and extra-cellular matrix, also called interstitial space. Glucose, oxygen, and other chemicals are delivered by the blood into this matrix. Cellular wastes must also travel though this matrix back to the bloodstream to be picked up and carried away.

A good analogy for this transport and delivery system is a community of people who get their food from the train. Trucks pick up the food from the train and deliver the food to the people. The trucks then pick up the wastes from the people of the town and transport them back to the train to be taken away. What would happen if the railroad that the train traveled on was congested with trash so the train couldn't move very fast? What if the streets were blocked and the trucks could barely get through? The people would be hungry and their homes would be accumulating garbage.

The train is analogous to a capillary that carries the blood to the tissue. The tissue is the community made up of cells that are the town's residents. The streets that the trucks drive on are analogous to the extra-cellular matrix that makes up the space between the cells. The average American who eats a processed diet has obstruction in his blood vessels, and the matrix is full of sludge. The cell membrane of a person who eats a high fat diet is stiff and inflexible; a lot of energy is used to pull in the nutrients and push out the wastes. This assumes the nutrition can even get to the cells through the matrix.

Metabolic wastes are produced when a cell is forever working and breaking down chemistries. However, when the garbage men can't get through the congested matrix, the cell's cleansing activities must slow down. Also, if the blood stream is clogged, the matrix congested and the cell membrane stiff; water, nutrients and oxygen are slow to get to the cell. Thus you have a toxic, hungry, and dehydrated cell. Hungry, thirsty, toxic cells translate to a hungry, thirsty, toxic organ. Since your body is made up of organs, your entire physical being is malnourished, dehydrated and toxic.

Disease preys on a weak body. This is why instead of treating disease, I suggest strengthening the body by feeding it energetic foods. Once the body regains normal function it will have the energy to cleanse and heal on its own. This has been proven for thousands of years with millions of people. I prefer to trust ancient "real life" experience over a recent experiment done on lab rats with fixed variables. Since when does a human live in a cage with all variables fixed? When you find one, let me know!

Cells respond to their environment by compensating. This is why most people do not feel the effects of their "poison habits" right away. When all the organs are depleted, the exhausted person has strong cravings and is irritable. You feel the way your cells feel. So what is the answer to all this?

Most people choose drugs or stimulants to get them through the day. Simply put, you've taken a cattle prod to your weak cells, forcing them into faster degeneration. Understanding how your cells work is the first step towards taking care of yourself. A lot of it is common sense. In speaking to the mind, the cells of the body are your internal children. You must feed them, give them water, and re-lay positive messages. Would you ever starve your outer children or deprive them of water? Would you ever choose not to bathe them and not keep them clean? Of course not!

So let's get bigger, shall we?

# Chapter Three

# Your Organs

*This network of Organs and Substances sustains the body activities of storing and spreading, preserving and transforming, absorbing and eliminating, ascending and descending, activating and quieting.*

—Ted Kaptchuk, O.M.D.

In the previous chapter we discussed an individual cell. Tissues contain millions of cells which are then formed into organs. Depending on the tissue to which they belong, the cells of a particular organ such as the kidney have a specific purpose. The functions of a kidney cell are entirely different from those of a cardiac cell. The kidney cell is specialized to filter blood and the cardiac cell is specialized to pump blood. These two cells look different and need different raw materials in order to perform their activities.

Organs that have similar functions are grouped together, constituting an organ system. An example of an organ system is the gastrointestinal system, whose organs perform the functions of digestion, absorption and elimination. These organs include the stomach, intestines, liver, gallbladder and pancreas.

Our bodies have five organ systems: the endocrine, digestive, respiratory, circulatory and immune systems. It is important that these systems are in communication and balance with one another. When they are functioning harmoniously, the body is able to execute the will of the mind.

The Chinese looked to nature to find out how the body worked. They observed the climate, rivers, streams, mountains and hills and used nature's landscape to describe the inner processes of the body.

The theory of the five elements was born in China in the 16th century-221 B.C. The five elements of water, fire, earth, metal and wood were used to explain all phenomena in the natural world and were considered to be indispensable. In *A Collection of Ancient Works* it is said, "Food relies on water and fire. Production relies on metal and wood. Earth gives birth to everything. They are used by the people." Each of the five elements are said to govern one or more organs of the body.

In addition to the five elements, the Chinese observed five seasons, believing the body was affected by weather.

The five seasons are spring, summer, late summer, autumn, and winter. When pertaining to the body, each of the five seasons corresponds to one of the five organ systems. The five seasons are also related to how we get results in life and adapt to its changing seasons. It is important to note that you have internal seasons that you cycle through for the duration of your life.

*Spring* is a time to grow and create new ideas, relationships, or life work. It is time to begin anew with a fresh green viewpoint on life. Spring gives way to *summer*, a time of activity and play. In the sunny yellow season you take the idea from spring and put it into action, allowing it to flourish and mature. In the season of *late summer* it is time to bear the fruit of our actions as the earth bears its fruit from planted seeds. It is a time of celebration and balance. *Autumn*, the next season, is a time of release. Just as the trees shed their leaves, we must let go of our mental baggage, as well as the clutter around the house. Autumn is a period of retrospection and cleansing. If we insist on holding on to sentimental things or relationships, we will experience anxiety and sadness. The *winter* is a cool quiet time. In the winter we must control our inner climate (emotions) in order to preserve our energy. In this season it is time for rest and inner work.

As mentioned before, each of the five elements (fire, earth, metal, water, and wood) governs one or more organs of the body. To keep it simple we will relate each element to one of the five major organ systems mentioned above (endocrine, digestive/eliminative, respiratory, circulatory and immune systems).

Let's start with the element *wood*. The wood governs the liver and gall bladder and represents the season of spring. It also governs the immune system, since it is tough in the face of adversity, such as illness. Wood pertains to the out-stretching, growing parts, which are the trees in nature; and in humans are the ligaments, tendons and muscles.

The liver, one of the most important organs in the body, suffers a great deal because of our stressful lifestyle. The liver stores the blood and is responsible for the "free flow of *Qi*." Every organ of the body needs *Qi* and blood; therefore, the liver is metaphorically called "the general of the army" by the *Nei Ching*, or classic textbook of Traditional Chinese Medicine.

The liver is closely related to our emotional activity. Prolonged mental irritation leads to liver dysfunction. For example, stagnated liver *Qi* is related to depression and fatigue. In contrast, hyperactive liver *Qi* is expressed in anger, insomnia and dizziness. In this way our emotions and the health of our liver are intertwined.

Eastern medicine connects the mind to organ functions. According to Elson M. Haas, M.D., the liver has much to do with the soul and the way you view life. A person who is enthusiastic about her vision has healthy and free flowing liver *Qi*. She is creative with a lot of ideas. Spring is a great time to conjure up an exciting new idea. It is the season associated with the wood element. A person with free flowing *Qi* directed by a healthy liver is a "free and easy wonderer" with pain-free flexible joints and freely moving muscles. A person who does not feel that spark for life may have deficient liver *Qi* or stagnated *Qi*.

Physiologically, the liver has over 500 jobs to do. The liver secretes bile which aids the digestive organs in absorbing nutrients. People who eat a diet high in mucus forming foods such as meat and dairy have thick bile which stagnates into gall stones. Rather than having the gall bladder removed, one could avoid foods that leave a slimy residue; instead, eat cleansing foods that clear the organs of stagnated waste.

Another major function of the liver is to store excess glucose or sugar in the form of glycogen. Glycogen is formed in the liver by mixing two pounds of sugar with four pounds of water. When blood sugar gets low, the liver and muscle cells start to break down glycogen into glucose. An adult has sufficient glycogen stored to provide enough energy for a normal day's activity. When that total supply must be used to feed the cells, the body will start to break down fat and protein in order to get the glucose it needs to live. Did you know that your brain needs a constant supply of glucose or else you will go into a coma or even die?

Glycogen, protein and fat are metabolized for energy when the cells are starving. This occurs when you are either fasting or on a low carbohydrate diet. Carbohydrates are necessary for the energy factories of the cells to run. They are the kindling that makes the fire burn in the energy factories. The more carbohydrates that are available to burn, the larger the fire. A large fire will burn fat logs. Therefore, according to basic biochemistry, you need carbohydrates to burn fat. Now you can understand why low carbohydrate diets do not work, and in fact are dangerous to one's health. The weight loss in the beginning is due to metabolism of glycogen (which stores water) and fats for energy. However, no one can stay on this starvation plan forever. Eventually you start eating carbohydrates again. The thyroid gland which runs the overall metabolic rate of the body is thrown off by the low carbohydrate diet and compensates by slowing down your metabolism. So when you start eating normally again, you will gain more fat than you originally had, due to the lower metabolic rate.

In addition to sugar, the liver breaks down cholesterol and fats. Excess hydrogenated fats and empty sugars are useless to the body, and cause the liver to become fatty and sluggish. A sluggish liver is ineffective in releasing the stored vitamins necessary for many functions of the body, including digestion. A person who gets sleepy after meals, regardless of what he eats, certainly has a sluggish liver. Between meals, it is the job of the liver to release stored glucose to keep the blood sugar from dropping too low. A person who suffers from hypoglycemia might want to pay more attention to what the liver needs in order to work properly.

The liver exists to detoxify normal cellular breakdown. In our current society, the liver is forced to carry a much higher burden than it is meant to bear. Yet with all that is dumped into the liver and the injurious food we choose to eat, it chugs away day after day without rest. The liver needs water, food and oxygen just as you do, in order to carry out its purpose in life. When this critical organ is nourished and hydrated, your emotions will lift and stabilize, the constant fatigue will go away and food will flow smoothly through your system.

The gall bladder is the other wood organ; it stores bile. This organ is absolutely necessary for proper digestion and should not be routinely removed. It is so simple to resolve gall stones when we use common sense. Liquefy the bile and the stones will dissolve.

The immune system is a delicate and organized community of armies. To remain balanced, i.e., neither deficient nor hyperactive, requires that its internal environment is fairly clean and stable. Whether you have autoimmune disease or a chronic infection makes little difference when you nourish the body with balancing foods and facilitate daily cleansing and elimination.

The next element, *fire*, is dominant in the season of summer. In relation to your internal seasons, the ideas that come up in the spring are acted upon in the summer. Fire governs the heart, the endocrine system and the small intestine. It is active, bright and full of heat. In *Miraculous Pivot*, another classic work of Traditional Chinese Medicine, it states, "The heart dominates vessels and the vessels house mind."

Through your heart you can access your intuition. First you must breathe, opening up the chest and quieting the ever-active thinking mind, so as to allow the soft voice of the spirit to come through. When there is an imbalance in the fire element, the person may be forgetful or have excessive dreams. They feel sadness rather than joy. Joy is the natural emotion of the heart.

The heart distributes blood to all the organs through its pumping actions. This "ruler" of organs pumps out five liters of blood per minute to be distributed to the 75 trillion cells via the vessel system. Strong emotions affect the pulse of the heart and the blood pressure inside the vessels; hence emotions affect all the organs through the heart and vessels.

When there is resistance in the vessel system due to a congestive diet high in fats, the heart must expend more energy in order to maintain sufficient blood flow. In response to the increased demand for stronger contractions, the heart enlarges, yet the muscle remains weak. It is difficult to get nutrients and oxygen to an enlarged heart through its tiny coronary arteries, especially when these arteries are filled with hard fat. Symptoms of any heart problem include fatigue, dizziness and depression. When the vessels are clear, distribution of oxygen and food to all the cells is free-flowing and efficient. The person as a whole is warm, nourished and oxygenated. Feeling internally warm and nourished, she spreads joy to others.

Another element governed by the fire element is the small intestine, a long tubular organ whose energy meridian goes to the top of the head where it influences the pituitary gland, otherwise known as the "master gland." Because of the energetic connection with the master gland, the small intestine affects the entire endocrine system.

The main function of the small intestine is to separate the "pure from the impure." It extracts the beneficial nutrients from the food and sends the rest to the colon. If the small intestine is healthy, it can absorb the nutrients your body needs. However in most people, a mucous layer referred to as mucoid plaque lines the intestines, making absorption of nutrients practically impossible. In addition to mal-absorption of vital nutrients, the putrid wastes which comprise the mucoid plaque, add to the toxic load of the liver and burden the immune system.

The Chinese believe that a sick digestive system is the culprit in most diseases. That is why they spent thousands of years studying plant foods, learning which ones nourish each organ. They incorporated the Five Element Theory into their daily meals by balancing each meal with foods that represent the five flavors and colors that correspond to each of the five elements. Therefore, the Chinese eat a wide variety of plants of all five flavors and colors.

A plant based diet does not leave residue in the body and facilitates proper absorption of nutrients and detoxification of waste. Doesn't it make sense that if you could absorb your food and eliminate wastes freely, you would feel open and light rather than bound up and congested?

The *earth* element governs the spleen and stomach and rules in the late summer. The stomach is called the "sea of food and fluid." The *Qi* of the stomach moves downward, so if this movement is impaired, the person may experience reflux, nausea or vomiting. The stomach extracts the earthly or postnatal essence of the food and water, passing it on to the spleen to be transformed and transported to the rest of the body.

Physiologically the food digested by the stomach moves downward to the small intestine where absorption of nutrients takes place.

The digestive system is very sensitive to changes in the nervous system. Apprehension, worry or obsessive thoughts disrupt digestion and you may get constipated from holding on to negativity. In contrast, an agitated, irritated nervous system causes the gut to rapidly expel its contents in the form of diarrhea. The stomach and spleen reside in the center of the body and the earth element invites you to relax and be centered. Lying down on the earth and allowing it to fully support you, permits you to release all your worries. Hugging a tree also provides a sense of earthly support and centeredness.

According to the Chinese, the spleen is the main digestive organ. Its energy is ascending (moves upward). The spleen takes the essence extracted by the stomach and transforms it into nutrient substance. The nutrient substance is transported to the lungs where it mixes with air and spreads to the rest of the body in the form of *Qi* and blood. The spleen is seen as the maker of *Qi* and blood, and according to the *Nei Ching*, "The five viscera all desire their breath of life from the spleen."

The spleen also metabolizes and spreads water throughout the body. It is responsible for ensuring that the tissues are moistened but not too damp. Dampness is seen as having edema, mucous and retained fluid. Did you know that the stomach can hold up to 20 liters of water? Your body should be about 70% water, the same ratio as for plant life and the earth. Most of the total body fluid, approximately two-thirds, should be retained inside the cell. One-third is outside the cell and one-fifth of that is retained in the vessels as plasma.

The body can retain up to 90 pounds of excess fluid in the tissues when the water metabolizing organs are weak or overburdened. The blood and lymph system can become so congested with residue-laden fluids that their vacuuming function will be inefficient. The water sits in the body like a stagnant pond, spawning the growth of fungus and bacteria. The physiological process just described conforms to Bechamp's belief that bacteria is formed from within the body.

The flavor associated with the spleen is sweet. It is interesting to note that as a result of consuming herbal food combinations that include the five flavors and five colors, my patients no longer struggle with cravings for unhealthy foods or stimulants. They simply start eating the Chinese herbal foods and the sweet cravings are gone within a week. This is certainly due in part to the balancing of the spleen *Qi*.

The next element is *metal*, which rules the organs of the respiratory system. Autumn, the season for letting go, belongs to this element. The respiratory system concerns itself with the breathing in and out of things. Through expiring we release toxins such as carbon dioxide and limiting thoughts. We have the choice to focus on what is great about our life or we can focus on what's not working for us. The only constant in life and in nature is change and if we resist change or hold on to things, we experience tightness in the lungs. By resisting change we may experience grief, which is the emotion of the lungs. I have observed lung ailments that began at the time someone experienced the loss of a loved one. When you do not mentally cleanse, the organs take up the unprocessed emotions and express them through physical symptoms.

"The lung rules $Qi$." In the lungs the $Qi$ from the nutrient substance extracted by the spleen mixes with the $Qi$ from the air and the resultant lung $Qi$ is dispersed throughout the body. Lung $Qi$ plays a role in the protective radiant shield that guards the body against "External Pernicious Influences."

The lung meridian is connected to the large intestine meridian; an imbalance of one affects the other. A congested colon will cause mucus to ascend into the lungs and sinuses. When the intestines are toxic and overburdened, the lungs become a garbage disposal, expelling more waste through the breath than normal. Mucus, which is used to carry waste material out of the body, begins to accumulate. Did you know that it takes a pint of mucous to carry out ¼ teaspoon of acid? Often in cleansing, people experience a lot of mucous, because the intestines aren't strong enough to eliminate the accumulated waste.

The lungs manifest onto the skin. Therefore, it is likely that an adult who currently suffers from eczema or dermatitis had allergies as a child. As just mentioned, the lungs are a backup to the colon. Accordingly, I have found that most adult acne is the result of internal morbid material coming from the overburdened colon. The body is so congested, the toxic material starts coming out through the skin. Topical treatments are ineffective in the long term because the cause is not being addressed. On the contrary, the use of such treatments contribute to a more advanced disease state due to their suppressive effects.

Let's take a closer look at the colon, which is another organ that needs to let go on a regular basis. Have you noticed that when you hold on to things or become mentally tight, the colon "holds on and won't move forward"? The colon receives unabsorbed portions of food from the small intestine to be expelled. As the feces move through the colon, water and electrolytes are reabsorbed through the colon membrane. Did you know that 80% of the water you drink is reabsorbed back into your body?

The intestinal lining is supposed to be around 2½ inches in diameter. More commonly, this lining gets expanded up to 12 inches in diameter to compensate for the accumulation of rotting food that never got digested. Professor Ehret, author of *Rational Fasting* and *Mucusless Diet*, wrote, "The vast majority of conditions of impaired health are due to accumulated poisons and excessive mucus within the body, which restrict proper functioning both chemically and mechanically." No wonder so many people suffer from allergies, asthma, skin outbreaks and many other similar ailments! These are outward expressions of the body's attempt to excrete poisons through vicarious means.

The element *water*, which rules in the winter, governs the water balancing organs. As mentioned earlier, the earth is approximately 70% water, as is the plant and the human body. Proper water metabolism is critical in order to hydrate the cells, lubricate the organs and keep the blood flowing. Organ systems that correspond to the water element include the kidneys, the adrenal glands and the reproductive organs.

The adrenal glands (or what the Chinese refer to as the kidneys) store the prenatal essence, which is our inherited energy. However, it is the "acquired essence," which comes from our lifestyle that mostly determines our state of health.

As the container of essence or *Jing*, the kidneys dominate the maturation and aging process. The kidney is known as the "root of *Qi*." Kidney essence manifests onto the hair. As kidney *Qi* declines, the hair turns white and falls out. Premature hair loss implies depleted kidney essence. Kidney essence also nourishes the marrow in the bones. Strong teeth reflect a surplus of marrow; therefore essence is plentiful. There are two kinds of marrow: bone and spinal. Spinal marrow connects to the brain. Since kidney essence nourishes the marrow, it also nourishes the brain. In *The Miraculous Pivot*, the Chinese describe the brain as "the sea of marrow"; hence, the kidneys play a key role in maintaining mental clarity.

In the role of fluid or water metabolism, the kidneys receive the impure essence from the lungs and further separate the clear from the turbid. It sends the turbid down to the bladder to be eliminated. This relates to the western view of the kidneys in that they filter the blood, sending the liquid wastes down to the bladder and reabsorbing the pure elements such as trace minerals, amino acids, and glucose. The entire plasma volume (2.75 liters) is filtered by the kidneys about 65 times per day. As such, urine is seen as a reflection of plasma.

The filtering action of the kidneys is critical to maintaining a certain blood pH. In particular, the presence of ions such as sodium and potassium in the blood depends on the ability of the kidneys to retain such crucial elements. Deficient kidney function or a reduced filtration rate results in edema or high blood pressure.

It is worth noting that the reproductive organs are ruled by the kidneys. Sexual impotence in males and frigidity in females are viewed as deficient kidney *Jing* by the Chinese doctor. By depositing more essence or live foods into your enzyme bank, you will find your youthful stamina renewed.

The emotion associated with the water element is fear. Fear is often felt by one who suffers from a urinary tract infection or other urinary dysfunctions, such as interstitial cystitis. The diagnosis of interstitial cystitis is a mysterious catch-all syndrome of the bladder which triggers immense pain. Passing kidney stones is also a frightening process. Negative thinking and a fearful outlook on life cause kidney dysfunction and deplete the *Jing*, resulting in premature aging and other water element imbalances. Regular practices that facilitate introspection will help to keep this winter element in balance.

We have looked at the five elements and the organs to which they correspond. I have studied Chinese medicine for years and as a medical student I thought it to be too mystical. Today, as a result of my personal experience and that of my patients, I can no longer question its truth. The western view is anatomical and obtains its information from the parts of cadavers. The eastern perspective is energetic, gathering its theories from living things, whether they are the sun and moon or mountains and streams. From the Chinese standpoint the patient is whole, comprised of physical, spiritual, and energetic matter. Hence, the Chinese doctor considers the internal emotions vital to the proper functioning of all the organs of the body.

# Chapter Four

# Your Immune System

*The natural healing force within each one of us is the greatest force
in getting well.*

— Hippocrates

The Chinese describe our defense system as the "radiant energy shield" that circulates on the exterior of our body. The immune system depends upon an unimpeded blood supply, minerals from the earth such as zinc and copper, and vitality that can protect us from "pernicious influences." The Chinese believe that illness is the result of lowered resistance, which in turn is caused by physiological and emotional stress as well as insufficient nourishment. The eastern view that teaches responsibility for one's health conflicts with the western medical theory that views the body as a victim to external invaders such as bacteria and viruses. Henry Lindlahr, M.D. was a pioneer in the nature cure movement and is author of *Philosophy of Natural Therapeutics*. He wrote about a physician, Dr. Pottenkofer who demonstrated to his University of Vienna students that bacteria do not cause disease. Dr. Pottenkofer supported this theory by swallowing millions of live cholera bacilli. Aside from slight nausea, he did not get sick from the experiment. Dr. Rodermund, who is also mentioned in Lindlahr's book, smeared his body with the exudate of smallpox. Before he was arrested and quarantined he came into contact with hundreds of people. Neither he nor one person he encountered ever came down with smallpox.

Louis Pasteur, a French chemist, developed a theory in the mid-1800s that the cause of disease could be traced to specific microorganisms. Therefore, it was the job of science to identify the organism linked to each disease and kill it. This became known as the famous "germ theory." Pasteur's premise eventually superseded the nature cure theory, giving birth to current western treatments that are combative in nature.

Antoinne Bechamp, M.D., a professor at the University of Lille, discounted the germ theory from the outset, writing that "disease is born of us and in us and that is as it should be, because the life of man, and of every other creature, is no more delivered over to chance than the course of the stars." Many other physicians during Pasteur's time also opposed the germ theory, and like Rodermund, performed experiments to disprove it. Their voices fell on deaf ears, however.

Pasteur's germ theory gave birth to the idea of fighting pathogens in the form of vaccinations and antibiotics. It wasn't until he made his fortune that Pasteur himself recanted his own theory on his deathbed stating, "Terrain is everything; the germ is nothing."

The use of vaccinations and antibiotics depend on the viability of the germ theory. The current medical system treats the body as a victim and its internal terrain becomes the battlefield between good and evil. But as Antoinne Bechamp argued, "Bacteria do not cause disease, and therefore serums and vaccines can neither prevent nor cure disease."

Rats live on garbage; as such, their food consists of decaying matter. Rats do not invade a clean city with a healthy sanitation system. The historic plagues of yellow fever, cholera and the bubonic plague that ravaged large populations did not go away because of vaccinations, since they did not yet exist! They disappeared when sanitation systems were introduced into the cities where people had been living in their wastes. Before this, there had been no plumbing, drainage, or ventilation, all of which contributed to the breeding of pathogens such as cholera that lived on morbid waste.

When the body is overloaded with debris and the bowels and kidneys are overworked; when a person's vitality is weak and blood abnormal, the accumulated morbid material must be excreted through vicarious methods of elimination such as the mucous membranes and skin. Abnormal processes of elimination are apparent due to symptoms of inflammation, such as fever, swelling, pain, runny nose and cough. What do you do when you get a cough and fever?

The plant's rootlets live in soil, which is the home of more microbes than anywhere else on earth. One teaspoon of dirt has more bacteria in it than all the animals and men that have ever existed. Likewise, the human body hosts more bacteria than the total count of its cells (75-100 trillion). Even if we were sterile inside, we are constantly exposed to the outside world of bacteria through open orifices such as the nose and mouth. This is what makes the germ theory and the ensuing medical system nonsensical. As E. Douglas Hume put it, "Had it not been for the mass selling of vaccines, Pasteur's germ theory of disease would have collapsed into obscurity."

In his book, *The Sanctity of Human Blood*, O'Shea quotes a 1985 statement by the International Association of Scientists and Biologicals: "Official data has shown that the large scale vaccinations undertaken in the U.S. have failed to obtain any significant improvement of the diseases for which they were supposed to provide immunization. In essence it was and is a failure." If that is the case, then why is the lifestream of a newborn invaded with a Hepatitis B virus? How about the mandatory measles vaccine if you want to go to college? This, despite the fact that a May 1996 article in the *Clinical Immunology and Pathology Journal* quoted a Center for Disease Control report stating that the measles vaccine "produces immune suppression, which contributes to an increased susceptibility to other infections." Why are the kids still getting vaccinated? Why are the soldiers of our military court marshaled if they refuse the mandatory vaccines, many of which are experimental? Unfortunately, the general public receives its education from television and other forms of controlled media and is kept in the dark about such matters.

At this point it would be wise to ask what your God-given immune system can do for you. Scientists accept that there are as many as 100 million different varieties of T-cells and 100 million antibodies patrolling the body. The immune system consists of several armies of defense that are specialized to kill specific germs. They are born in the bone marrow and many of them mature in your thymus gland, which resides in the upper middle chest. The immune system is just learning its ropes during the first two years of life. It matures by being exposed to different pathogens during the growing years. The armies learn through practice how to defend us by developing natural immunity to the microorganisms that we are exposed to as a child.

A diet high in mucus-forming foods such as meat and dairy, burdens the cells of the immune system. Undigested proteins from the intestines are absorbed into the bloodstream, to which the immune cells react by attaching antibodies. The foreign protein with an antibody attached is referred to as an antibody-antigen complex. This type of immune response is implicated in all sorts of allergies and ailments of immunodeficiency.

How can the immune system take care of business when all of its workers are busy digesting food? The more toxic the body, the harder the immune system has to work in order to protect the delicate balance of the blood. Autointoxication leads to immunodeficiency and allergies to food, animals and plants of nature. It is not natural to be allergic to anything of the earth. A hyperactive immune system that has been overworked for so long loses its ability to know the difference between natural and unnatural. Taken to a more degenerative state, the armies turn inward and can no longer distinguish self from non-self. Fibromyalgia, lupus, rheumatoid arthritis, Hashimoto's and multiple sclerosis are some of the modern day diagnoses for an immune system gone crazy.

So what is the true cause of disease? D.W. Cavanough, M.D., of Cornell University said, "There is only one major disease, and that is malnutrition. All ailments and afflictions are directly traceable to this disease. Food crops grown on depleted soil produce malnourished bodies and disease preys on malnourished bodies."

It is true that we all have at least one weak area or a disposition to manifest symptoms in a certain organ system. This weak disposition originated in the "sins" of our forbearers and was transferred through family members. By sins, I mean pathogenic lifestyles that weaken a particular organ system, and this weakness is transferred to the offspring. For example, my family's weaknesses are revealed through the nervous and digestive systems. Through lifestyle changes I have overcome my inherited weaknesses. One of my patients inherited psoriases that started at age 40. Every woman in her family has suffered with this weakness. Six months into my program, she had cleansed out all the psoric miasms and today remains free of psoriases. She has broken the chain of psoriases in her family, and if she were to have children, it is unlikely that she would pass on this trait.

It is possible for anyone to overcome inherited organ weakness by committing to a healthy lifestyle. In his book, *Nutrition and Physical Degeneration,* Dr. Weston Price documented his study of the effect of nutrition on a person's genes. He observed primitive natives around the world and noticed the effect of commercialized food on facial structure and dental health. Offspring of the parents who started eating the western diet were born with narrow faces and crowded teeth. What used to be a society known to have the healthiest teeth in the world is now one that is suffering from rampant tooth decay. In 1950, Royal Lee, M.D., stated: "Trace mineral deficiency, it is evident, can act also to impair hereditary transmission."

The late Josef Issels, M.D., a renowned cancer researcher and practitioner, refers to inherited predisposition as the prenatal cause of disease, while environmental factors make up the postnatal cause of disease. Environmental irritants are plentiful in today's industrialized society. Compounded with the fact that we are not getting the nutrients we need from our food, it is no wonder that cancer is the number one cause of death in this country. We are constantly exposed to heavy metals in the air, on food and in our water.

I disagree with the notion that if breast cancer runs in the family, you are at a higher risk and should get yearly mammograms (which exposes the breast tissue to radiation). It might be more accurate to say that the women belonging to that family inherited breast tissue that is not resilient to the onslaught of injurious substances. Fortunately you can affect whether or not you develop the disease by adjusting the environmental factors. Structurally, breast tissue contains a lot of draining lymph channels. Massaging the breasts upward towards the arm pits in combination with a pure natural diet minimizes the insults that this tissue must endure.

The relationship between food and disease is apparent and has been evidenced all over the world. Does the FDA exist to protect our food? Dr. Harvey Wiley, M.D., who founded the FDA, fought hard to prevent the adulteration of food through refining and processing. Sadly, Dr. Wiley was removed from office in 1912 and replaced by Elmer Nelson, M.D., who supported the profit-motivated interests of the food manufacturers. Ever since Wiley's removal from office, the American Food Machine has had the FDA in its pockets. Nelson was relentless in his testimonies to the courts that degenerative diseases are not the result of nutritional deficiencies.

How pure is our food today? Today's apples may have up to 36 chemicals on their outer surfaces. Food irradiation exposes food to the equivalent of 2.5 million chest x-rays. According to a report released by the FDA called Food Defect Action Levels, a 7-ounce glass of tomato juice can have up to 20 maggots of fly eggs (maggots); a one-pound box of macaroni can have up to nine rodent fragments; a one-pound box of frozen broccoli can have 276 aphids; 3.5 ounces of apple butter can have up to five whole insects; and one pound of cocoa beans can have up to ten milligrams of rodent feces.

It is well known that processed food contains additives that make you hungry and addicted to the food. It has also been proven that some of the additives even control how fast you eat. Are you aware of when you are eating your food too fast, barely chewing each bite? It all makes sense, because when you are excessively hungry and eat your food too quickly you will end up buying more food.

Sugar is the biggest culprit in today's adulterated foods. An article published in the *Well Being Journal* stated that studies show when people consume MSG-containing foods, they eat faster. Sugar substance, whether in the form of white sugar, high fructose corn syrup or MSG, is highly addictive and suppresses the immune system. Eight teaspoons of sugar (one can of soda) suppress the immune system by 25% for 12 hours. Twelve teaspoons of sugar suppress the immune system by 95% for 12 hours. The average American consumes 53 teaspoons of sugar per day. By living on food that is full of calories and devoid of vitamins and minerals, you are starving yourself to the death bed, all the while having food in your stomach.

Let's talk about cancer, an immunodeficiency disease, and the number one cause of death in the United States. We declared "war" on cancer in 1971. As of 1970, 17.2% of all deaths were from cancer. Today, according to the American Cancer Society's journal, *A Cancer Journal for Clinicians*, North Americans suffer the highest incidence of cancer of any region in the world. Yet we spend more money than any other nation on cancer research, billions of dollars per year. Where is all this money going? The research money goes to new and improved chemotherapy and radiation treatments, the two main therapies for cancer in mainstream medicine, and also known to cause cancer. Thirty-four years into the "war on cancer," it is now the number one cause of death. Chemotherapy and radiation are not working but appear instead to be worsening the problem. When asked why they keep using these therapies, a cancer research expert answered, "because they don't know what else to do."

Left to the scientific community, doomsday will be knocking at your door unless you decide to take on your health the way you take on other seemingly important areas of your life. The body you were given is the only house you'll live in for the rest of your life. If you take care of it only half as well as you take care of your outer house, you will be one of the healthiest people you know.

The first step in taking back your health is to understand how the body uses energy. The body must prioritize its functions due to the limited amount of energy it has, depending on whether we are replenishing our essence or depleting it. There are seven main priorities. The first priority is to take care of the **crucial functions**, which include the heart and lungs. The second priority is taking care of the **muscles**, since the heart is a muscle and our digestive system depends on muscular function to propel food through the intestines. Did you know that skeletal muscle contraction is required just to sit in a chair?

The third priority is **cleansing**. The main cleansing organs of your body are the liver, kidney and intestines. When these guys are overburdened due to heavy foods, acidic waste starts to accumulate. Lack of nourishment and dehydration compound the problem because the cleansing organs become weaker and more sluggish in their functions. The vessel system, including the lymph channels, is responsible for clearing waste from the tissues and transporting it to the liver to be neutralized. However, when the vessel system gets overloaded due to sluggish detoxification and elimination, the waste remains in the tissues. The blood continues to deposit residue into the tissues to preserve its strict pH of 7.4. The body cells and tissues work optimally at a pH close to that of the blood; however they can still survive at a more acidic pH all the way down to 3. On the contrary, if the blood stream pH alters even slightly, death can ensue. This process of robbing Peter to Save Paul is what goes on in your body every day until you lighten up the diet and add some more nourishment. Drinking more water is also necessary if you want to start moving the debris out of your cells.

What does all of this mean in lay person's terms? The symptoms you complain about are coming from irritated tissues and cells. Doctors do blood tests to catch disease. However, there is so much going on in the tissues of your body that a blood test will not catch. If you are relying on blood tests you are waiting too long to catch disease. So many people come to me because they are not getting answers from their medical doctors. They are frustrated and weary of being told that nothing's wrong when in fact, their bodies and organ systems are telling them they're not performing optimally—so they know there must be a problem somewhere. They continue to pay for more office visits only to hear the doctor tell them their blood tests are normal, which means "nothing's wrong." By the time something shows up on a blood test, the problem has been in the body tissues for a very long time, and the excess toxins and fats are now distressing the blood. Then, if we follow through with the western medical model, we're intimidated into taking drugs or getting something cut out. Prevention through right living and education is the only way out of this cycle called damage control.

The fourth priority of the body is **fat maintenance**. Fat tissue is a safe place to store toxins; therefore, if your diet leaves noxious residue in the body, you will not be lean no matter how much you exercise. The body is naturally lean. However, if it's a choice to be thin or survive in the midst of morbid waste, the body will choose life and hold onto fat to keep the chemicals away from the crucial organs and blood.

The fifth priority is the **immune system**. We talked about the immune system in terms of being deficient or hyperactive. Balance is the key to a vital immune system. As long as the internal environment is clean and strong, the immune system will have sufficient energy to fight off foreign pathogens as they enter the body.

The sixth priority is **regeneration**. The body you have today is not the same you had a year ago. Most people are degenerating as they age. In ancient times, the Chinese pursued regeneration as they grew older, paying doctors to keep them healthy. They believed that the period from age 21 to 150 was for physical regeneration, and they were active until the day they died. This explains the investment of thousands of years in the study of plants and inner work in order to achieve optimal health and higher mind.

The seventh priority is **higher mind**. Over 50% of American women take a pill to be happy. This doesn't include all the men and women who silently suffer day in and day out. They believe they don't have a choice because that's what their doctor told them. Hopefully after reading this book you will conclude that depression is an energy crisis problem and you *can* make a different choice.

In his book, *Fit for Life*, Harvey Diamond identifies seven stages of degeneration that lead to cancer. Merely knowing the process of degeneration allows you to turn your health around by choosing to climb up through these stages back to health. The first stage of degeneration is **enervation**. When the body's detoxifying and eliminative organs become overworked and the body's essence is depleted due to over-expenditure and/or malnourishment, fatigue sets in. More naps and longer nights of sleep are needed. In addition to feeling sluggish, a decreased appetite is common during this stage. Energy is diverted from the high demands of the digestive system to the more urgent condition of toxic overload.

During this time, it is important to either fast or eat fruit, which is the easiest food to digest as your body recovers its equilibrium. Since most people are not aware that there is an energy crises going on in their body, they self-stimulate to keep up with the demands of their high-stress lifestyle. Coffee, cigarettes, sugar, meat and fatty foods kick start the body's stress organs and give us a thrill of energy. As we all know, there's a down side to this "high" that can occur as soon as after just a few minutes. The long term effect is a downward descent to the second step of degeneration called **toxemia**.

In toxemia, the morbid material accumulates in the lymph nodes and blood. Fever exemplifies this stage of disease. Fever is the body's attempt to increase enzyme activity and kill pathogens. What do you do when you get a fever? Whenever you suppress fever with ice or medication, you have forced the body into irritation, the third stage of disease.

**Irritation** is experienced when the nervous system becomes inundated with toxins. Anxiety, depression, flying off the handle, itchy skin, headaches and bad breath are some of the symptoms of irritation. Common band-aids used at this level of disease are antidepressants, sleeping pills, aspirin and pain medications. People live for years with these symptoms, while suppressing the body's many cries for proper nutrition and emotional balance. As long as you treat the symptoms, the prolonged irritation leads to inflammation, the fourth stage of degeneration.

**Inflammation** is the body's most energetic attempt to expel toxins. Heat, pain, swelling and any "itis" syndrome is characteristic of this degenerative stage. The areas of the body in which toxins are concentrated become inflamed, such as in swollen lymph nodes, eczema, or psoriasis. Whenever you treat the symptoms of inflammation with ice or medications such as steroids and anti-inflammatories, you have forced the body into the fifth stage of disease, called **ulceration**. The body has been under assault for so long, vast amounts of tissues continue to be destroyed by pathogenic material. Just like a city filled with garbage is overrun by rats, a body filled with morbid waste is overrun by pathogens.

The sixth stage marks **induration** in which the body lays down fibrous tissue to replace the dying organ tissue. The areas of accumulated debris become hardened. Cysts, fibroids and benign tumors are often sub-clinical and by the time they're picked up by a standard diagnostic exam such as ultrasound, they have been there for years. When the diseased cells become so engorged with poison, they "go crazy" and start to divide uncontrollably into cells that have no purpose or biological function. This tumor is cut off from the messages from the brain and escapes the immune system's vigilance. The diagnosis of **cancer** identifies the seventh stage of disease and is the final attempt by the body to survive in its own morbid waste.

I know what the cure for cancer is and it doesn't cost a dime. It is your body! No doctor, no drug, and no supplement or food item can cure you. Your body developed the symptom of cancer so that you could live, despite your poor choices. At any time, you can befriend your body and start climbing those stairs towards optimal health. Be aware, however, that as you climb you will move through the stages of disease just mentioned and experience many of the symptoms of each stage. It is important to not suppress these symptoms of cleansing, but instead to facilitate the body's progress toward health. You will know that you are regenerating when you look and feel younger than you did a month or year ago. Healing time will depend on how much regeneration needs to be done in order to bring your organ systems into balance. Be patient. It took a long time to get to where you are now, so don't expect anything to happen overnight!

On this journey to optimal health you choose to no longer treat symptoms, so when you experience discomfort while you're going through the cleansing process, be grateful that your body has the energy to expel toxins. Eat lightly and drink lots of fluid, for nothing withstands a flood. As hardened diseased tissue is broken down and removed, flushing it out with water will make your cleansing experience much more comfortable. It will also eliminate the chance of reabsorbing into the blood what was just pulled out. Like nature, your body works in its own time, so I cannot emphasize enough that patience is truly a virtue.

## Chapter Five

# Your Digestive/Eliminative System

*Teach me Thy way, O Lord; and lead me in a plain path...*

—Psalms 97:11

Eating is the act of choosing your fuel with education and consciousness, and it starts with your mouth. Chewing your food is the first step in digestion. Human saliva contains the enzyme ptyalin which begins the breakdown of starch into simple sugars. The food is propelled down the esophagus, a muscular tube, to be further broken down in the stomach. Very little digestion takes place in the upper stomach. It is here that food, containing its own active enzymes, will start to digest itself. Unfortunately, the common diet of devitalized food has no enzymes and sits fermenting in the cardiac portion of the stomach. This is where reflux disease comes in.

The medical system believes it is your own stomach acid that causes reflux disease. In reality the reflux is there as a result of the presence of organic acids of putrefaction and fermentation, produced by the stagnant indigestible food. As soon as a person changes their diet to foods that are digestible, the reflux goes away.

Eventually the food moves down to the lower portion of the stomach where hydrochloric acid and pepsin start the process of breaking down proteins. The length of time that food sits in the stomach depends on its type. For example, carbohydrates move through much faster than a high protein meal because we have more enzymes for breaking down starch than we do protein. That's why a high protein, high fat meal provides a longer satiation time than a meal high in complex carbohydrates, such as rice and vegetables. People will say that the fatty meal "stuck to their ribs." This feeling of a full stomach is not what you want. It is not healthy to have undigested food sitting in the stomach for hours and hours putrefying, thus providing fuel for pathogenic bacteria such as H.pylori.

H.pylori has been identified to cause ulcers. However, this bug is a part of our normal flora in low counts. It is only when we feed it garbage that it becomes pathogenic and overgrows. This is an example of the terrain theory, which states that the bugs are the effect and not the cause of diseased tissue. The original cause of ulcers is the presence of morbid material that weakens the cells of the body, lowering their resistance. In addition, the decaying material provides food to the potentially harmful bacteria. Accordingly, it is ineffective to treat the bug with an antibiotic and then take an antacid to inhibit hydrochloric acid secretions, which are needed to digest proteins and kill bacteria. Reflux disease affects sixty-one million Americans, and the medications are clearly not working. In addition to exacerbating the reflux disease, acid blockers inhibit mineral absorption. Given that digestive enzymes depend on minerals to work, this propagates the indigestion problem that causes the reflux in the first place.

A hiatal hernia is the end result of spastic contractions of the stomach mucosa in response to food-borne acids. The body creates a hernia in order to protect itself from the acids being released from the spoiled food. Treating the hernia is not the answer. Removing the indigestible food from one's diet will offer great relief. To have a healthy stomach, the mucosa needs to be intact and the secretion glands need nourishment so they can function optimally.

Any obstacles that are blocking the ability for the body to heal itself must be removed from the diet. The number one stomach-buster is caffeine. Caffeine is also harmful to the liver, kidneys and adrenal glands. Soda pop is so acidic, a 16-ounce bottle would need to be diluted with 10 gallons of water to bring its pH up to 7.3, the pH of blood. Other major stomach-busters include sugar, preservatives, alcohol and chocolate.

Once the food is partially digested by the stomach and is ready to enter the small intestine, it is called *chyme*. The chyme passes through a valve called the pyloric sphincter to the small intestine, which is a 22-foot long coiled tube. Finger-like projections called *villi* line the intestinal walls. The presence of villi, in addition to a carpet-like brush border, give the small intestines an actual length of 200 square feet. It is here that 90% of the absorption of food into the bloodstream takes place.

Up to this point, the food has not actually been inside the body proper. Until the food is absorbed through the lining of the small intestine, it is separated by the mucosal walls of the mouth, esophagus, and stomach. This is a protective mechanism for the body. Fifty percent of your immune system is along your digestive tract. The barrier of the tract and friendly bacteria serve to protect the rest of your body from the food until it has been completely broken down and purified. Of course this is in an ideal situation in which the intestinal lining is healthy and the friendly bacteria are thriving. Realistically, the majority of Americans have leaky intestines and sparse friendly bacteria, leaving the rest of the body vulnerable to the invasion of undigested proteins and foreign bacteria.

Digestion continues in the small intestine, involving the secretions of the pancreas and gall bladder. The acidic chyme is neutralized by the alkaline secretions of the duodenum (the first part of the small intestine). The presence of fat in the duodenum stimulates the gallbladder to release stored bile that is manufactured by the liver. Bile acids serve as our body's detergents by emulsifying the fats in our foods. The fatty acids in the small intestine are absorbed into lacteals, which lead into the lymph system.

In the small intestine, proteins are broken down into amino acids and carbohydrates are broken down into monosaccharides. Vitamins and minerals are absorbed in their original state. These micronutrients will now pass into the blood stream to feed the rest of the body.

Micronutrients are not the only substances formed during the process of digestion. Highly toxic biogenic amines and ptomaines are also formed and although highly toxic, do not injure the body, as detoxification systems exist to make them harmless before they reach the bloodstream. First in the line of defense is the mucus membrane of the small intestine, which neutralizes these noxious agents. However, if the intestinal lining is damaged, the toxic chemicals will pass into the blood and must be broken down by the liver, our second detoxifying system. In today's industrialized society with over-consumption of injurious substances, the liver is burdened with the job of the small intestine. Inflamed intestines can no longer serve the function of protecting the blood from large foreign proteins and toxic byproducts of bacterial fermentation.

It is important to note that digestion depends on enzymes, vitamins, minerals and water. Minerals are necessary for enzyme function and are the only source of alkalinity for your body. The average diet is high in meat, dairy and other acidifying foods, which uses up the minerals and thus leads to decreased enzyme activity. If the food we eat does not contain its own enzymes, vitamins and minerals, the liver and adrenal glands must give up their stores of these nutrients in order for digestion of the devitalized food to continue. The end result for every lifeless meal is depletion instead of nourishment. In fact, one average American meal is equal to a day's hard labor on the body.

From the small intestine, the extracted micronutrients are transported to the liver through the bloodstream. The most complex organ of the body, the liver performs over 500 different functions every day. It is a manufacturing plant that takes the nutrient substances from the small intestine and builds proteins, carbohydrates and fats, in addition to many other nutrients that are needed throughout the body. The liver also forms vitamin A and stores it along with vitamins D and B-complex, and minerals such as copper, zinc, and iron. The liver deactivates all the hormones, thus influencing metabolism.

Detoxifying cells of the liver are loaded with mitochondria; these organelles are very sensitive to environmental toxins. As long as these little energy factories are getting enough nutrients and are not assaulted by harmful metals and pesticides, the liver can keep up with the high demands of today's lifestyle. In cases of malnutrition and toxic overload, the liver becomes sluggish from storage of acids, ammonia and other types of poisons. Other organs are now exposed to toxins and must store them until the liver regains normal function.

Hormone metabolism is affected when the liver suffers, leading to imbalances in the endocrine system. I wonder how often a thyroid imbalance medicated with a drug could have been corrected by cleaning up the liver. I have seen long-standing thyroid problems resolved simply from nourishing and cleansing the body. I have also read about many studies done on pre-menstrual syndrome (PMS) for new drugs. To this day, scientists still do not completely understand why women suffer from PMS. I have found that by nourishing, balancing and cleansing the liver, any hormone imbalance is easily resolved.

Within 8 to 10 hours of eating, the food has passed through the small intestine and enters the large intestine via the ileocecal valve. This valve is located in the lower right-hand side of your abdomen. The colon, a muscular tube, is about 6 feet long. The colon is shaped into pouches called *haustras*. These haustras allow for considerable expansion. The diameter of a healthy colon is 2 ½ inches. However in diseased colons, the membrane can stretch up to 12 inches in diameter. More than 400 species of friendly bacteria, weighing about 3 pounds in a normal colon, serve to keep bad bacteria in check. Their feeding processes produce vitamin K and some of the B vitamins.

Few sensory nerves innervate the colon. This is clinically relevant in that most people do not realize they have colon disease until it's too late. By the time a person with abdominal pain visits his gastroenterologist, the disease has progressed into its advanced stages.

Dr. Bernard Jensen traveled throughout the world studying the lifestyles of healthy cultures and learning from masters of longevity. At his sanitarium where he treated thousands of patients diagnosed with a wide variety of ailments, he focused on bowel health and became an expert in the workings of the digestive tract because he believed that disease originates in the decaying matter of weak and overburdened intestines. Dr. Jensen proved without a doubt that there is a direct relationship between the health of the bowels and the proper functioning of the rest of the body. With a healthy lifestyle, the bowels are revitalized, and long-standing noxious wastes are purged from the system. As a result of bowel revitalization and cleansing, Dr. Jensen witnessed the healing of many types of degenerative ailments.

A diet high in mucus forming meat, dairy, and other fiberless foods leaves behind a slimy coating. Dr. Tim O'Shea tells us of the experience of Dr. Harvey Kellogg, a noted surgeon in Michigan. Of the 22,000 operations that Dr. Kellogg personally performed, none of the colons was clean. Of the 100,000 operations that he supervised, Dr. Kellogg reported that only 6% of the colons did not have mucoid plaque. In the book, *Cleanse and Purify*, Dr. Richard Anderson spoke of a doctor he met who worked in the area of post-mortem diagnoses. This doctor, who worked with thousands of cadavers, spoke with Dr. Anderson about what he observed in the cadavers: "We see the mucoid plaque in everyone and have to blow the stuff right out of the intestines. In the filthy substance are all sorts of worms, bacteria, fungi, and many unidentifiable things."

Here's the tricky part. When the bowels are coated with this mucoid plaque, absorption of nutrients is impeded. People with sluggish bowels have a hard time committing themselves to a whole food diet because no matter how nutritive the food may be, they are not absorbing the essentials; hence, they notice little change in their overall state of health. Herbert Shelton wrote that people are not suffering from deficiency disease due to lack of food as much as they are suffering from faulty assimilation. Many who have tried eating a whole food diet said they felt more tired, even though they were eating healthily, because they no longer consumed the stimulating foods such as meat and coffee. In withdrawing from the drug foods, they face their true state of health without the mask of stimulants. Often as a result, they don't stay with the healthy diet and turn once again to their stimulants.

The answer to this perplexing problem is to *nourish and cleanse the cells of the intestines directly, at the source of the problem.* Then proper absorption of nutrients can take place and the vitality of the body will be restored. Fortunately, the cells of the digestive tract divide every 2-5 days, which means that when the conditions around those cells change, the stomach and small intestine recover quickly. The key is to provide nutrients that do not require any digestive effort so the digestive tract itself is provided with readily available fuel. This is accomplished through dehydrated and concentrated organ-specific food herbs that are free of chemical residue. When the essence of food is intact, the powerhouse of the intestines is recharged.

This is how I recovered my own optimal level of health. My digestive system was able to rest while receiving nourishment and I was then able to absorb nutrients and eliminate waste. Every aspect of my life—physical, mental and emotional—improved as a result!

One of the unhealthiest foods a human can eat is meat. Animal protein is very difficult for the human digestive system to break down. Our digestive tract bears a closer resemblance to that of a chimpanzee (a plant-eating animal) than a rat (a flesh-eating animal), yet most medical studies for the purpose of discovering more about the human body, are conducted on rats. A carnivore or flesh-eating animal has long, sharp, pointed teeth for ripping and chewing flesh. The human has molars for crushing and grinding vegetation. The saliva of a carnivore is acidic for digestion of animal protein. The saliva of humans is alkaline and contains ptyalin for digesting starch. The carnivore's stomach is a simple round sack that secretes 10 times more hydrochloric acid than the human stomach. The human stomach is oblong, complex and convoluted and has 10 times less hydrochloric acid than that of a carnivore. The intestines of a carnivore are 3 times the length of the trunk, designed for rapid expulsion of meat which rots quickly. The human intestines are 12 times the length of our trunks, designed for thorough extraction of nutrients.

A typical American eats 75 grams of protein per day. Since the stomach is not equipped to produce the amount of hydrochloric acid needed to break it down, the undigested animal protein moves into the small intestine. Part of the reason for this is that the protein chains are denatured during the cooking process, so the digestive enzymes do not recognize the shape of the food proteins.

A healthy transit time for movement of food through the digestive tract is 18 hours. This means from the time you put the food into your mouth and eliminate the waste from that food, 18 hours have passed. The average American has a transit time of 24 to 36 hours. Would you eat a steak if it sat on your kitchen counter for 18 hours at 99 degrees?

Meat rots and putrefies in the intestines, giving off sulphuric and phosphoric acids along with other harmful byproducts. Mucoproteins and toxic chemicals called *scatals*, get absorbed into the bloodstream and congest the liver. The immune system is called to action due to the presence of foreign agents in the blood. The adrenal glands are stimulated due to the high vitamin demands, in order to fuel more enzymes.

What are the clinical results of such a chain of events? Over-stimulated adrenal glands, an overactive immune system and a sluggish liver lead to ailments such as chronic fatigue, autoimmune diseases, immunodeficiencies, and liver disease. Whenever a substance stimulates an organ, there is a propensity to become addicted to that substance. This is why one sees so many people addicted to meat and dairy. These two and sugar are the three most addictive food groups. As if addiction and fatigue aren't enough, bugs also have a part to play in this storyline.

The purpose of fungus is to break down decaying matter. Remember the plant that lives harmoniously with fungus which grows along its rootlets? When the plant is weak, the fungus takes down the plant and returns it to the earth. When we have dead matter in our weakened gut, normal fungus becomes pathogenic because its whole purpose in life is to break down decaying matter. The friendly bacteria are consumed by the fungus, and the immune system fights relentlessly to control its growth. If the body is malnourished, there's no hope of overcoming this horrific process. Symptoms of *candidiases* or Candida Albicans are widespread and frustrating. The person may be tired, depressed, constipated and always hungry. Most likely they suffer from colitis, chronic skin outbreaks, allergies, autoimmune disease, and hormone imbalances.

Anatomical differences between humans and carnivores are just one reason why we shouldn't eat meat. The average meat eater absorbs 500 doses of antibiotics per year from the meat they consume. Your friendly bacteria don't have a chance to defend themselves against this onslaught. Decreased friendly bacteria means lowered resistance to Candida Albicans. The antibiotics in meat, in addition to the 3 million pounds administered to humans in the treatment of disease, are spawning a new era of intelligent viruses. In 1998, the *Journal of Science* called the meat industry "the driving force behind the development of antibiotic resistance in certain bacteria that cause human disease." My father, who lives in Oklahoma, told me about some cattle he saw that were literally standing in feces. They couldn't even lie down or they would be covered in their own waste. Approximately 1.6 billion tons of manure are produced each year by the cattle industry. It's all over the place and they can't keep it from getting into the meat itself.

In his book, *The Food Revolution*, John Robbins, M.D. did an excellent job revealing the truths about the U.S. food industry. At least the Europeans know better than to allow manure into their food by paying the U.S. government millions of dollars each year to keep our grotesque meat out of their countries.

Why do Americans eat so much meat, you may ask. Consider that our nutritional education has been paid for by three of the four food groups represented on the food pyramid. The American Dairy Association, the farming industry and the American Meat Association paid for our education in the schools and in the media. The meat and dairy associations capitalized on a study of rats conducted in 1914 by two research scientists, Osborn and Mendel, that proved (they claim) that animal protein is superior to vegetable protein. However, as I point out, rats and humans are completely different. Rat's breast milk is 49 percent protein and human breast milk is only 5 percent protein, yet a baby doubles his size in the first six months of life solely from mother's milk. The proposal that we need huge amounts of protein to grow bigger and stronger is not based on valid evidence. Those studies are paid for by the meat industry and are completely unrealistic. It is this commercialized idea that is killing most Americans today.

Let's look at what's real. The silverback gorilla, which is three times the size of man and 30 times stronger, is a raw vegetarian. All the beasts of burden are vegetarians. Professional athletes and bodybuilders are discovering new levels of energy by converting to vegetarian diets.

The idea that animal meat is the only source of complete protein also came from rat experiments and was capitalized on by the meat industry. The Food and Nutrition Board of the National Research Council states, "One of the biggest fallacies ever perpetuated is that there is any need for so-called 'complete protein'." Our bodies recycle 70% of the protein waste; hence we lose only about 23 grams of protein a day. To replenish this lost protein, your body needs only about 1.5 pounds of protein a month. Moreover, an amino acid pool is used by the body to extract the amino acids it needs, and the rest is saved for future use. Therefore, it is not necessary to consume all the amino acids in one sitting. The body is going to break up the proteins, use and store the amino acids as needed.

The China Health Project, known as the "grand prix of Epidemiology" and referred to as one of the most rigorous and conclusive studies in the history of health research, produced some interesting results. The traditional Chinese eat cleansing foods such as vegetables, grains and legumes, some fish and no dairy. They obtain 7% of their protein from animal products, and Americans obtain 70% of their protein from animals. The traditional Chinese consume 20% more calories than Americans but Americans are 25% fatter.

In contrast, urban areas of China that have adopted the foods of commerce into their lifestyles have also adopted the western diseases of diabetes, cancer and heart disease. The more rural areas of China that have kept to their traditions do not suffer from these diseases of excess.

Reports in the American Journal of Clinical Nutrition say that people do not need to consume more than 2.5% of their daily caloric intake from protein. The World Health Organization reports that we need no more than 4.5% of calories from protein. This translates to 25-35 grams of protein per day. Meanwhile the average American eats 75-100 grams of protein a day – 5 times the actual need. How many calories are provided from protein in raw fruits and vegetables? Spinach is 49% protein, broccoli is 45% protein, and bananas are 5% protein. Bananas, apples, and carrots are three examples of plant foods that supply all 8 essential amino acids, thereby meeting the definition of a complete protein.

Concerning protein consumption and degenerative diseases, T. Colin Campbell, a professor of Nutritional Sciences at Cornell University and senior science advisor to the American Institute for Cancer Research, says there is "a strong correlation between dietary protein intake and cancer of the breast, prostate, pancreas and colon." Likewise, Myron Winick, director of Columbia University's Institute of Human Nutrition, has found strong evidence of "a relationship between high-protein diets and cancer of the colon."

In a report in the October 9, 2001 issue of the journal *Circulation*, the Nutrition Committee of the American Heart Association wrote, "High-protein diets may also be associated with increased risk for coronary heart disease due to intakes of saturated fat, cholesterol and other associated dietary factors . . . high-protein diets are not recommended because they restrict healthful foods that provide essential nutrients and do not provide the variety of foods needed to adequately meet nutritional needs. Individuals who follow these diets are therefore at risk for compromised vitamin and mineral intake, as well as potential cardiac, renal, bone, and liver abnormalities overall." It seems that the scientific community is not behind the high protein fad diets.

What is it going to take for us to give up our drug foods and turn to nature for healing? *There is one way to turn your health around, and achieve those high levels of optimal function.* Regardless of how hopeless it may seem, **start to feed the interdependent organ systems nutrient dense food that is loaded with phytonutrients and alive with enzymes.** These foods in addition to **a lot of fiber,** which literally pulls the sticky slime from the intestinal walls, will regenerate the entire digestive system. The immune system will no longer have to engage its armies with every meal you eat, and can attend to its normal battles. Where there is healthy vibrant tissue, efficient detoxifying systems and a powerful immune system, no fungus or any other pathogen can survive.

I have personally found that by feeding the body a wide variety of plant foods that are readily available to the digestive system, cravings disappear. We are hungry and overeat because we are malnourished, due to nutrient deficiencies and poor assimilation. We crave sugar due to a spleen imbalance that is caused by depriving ourselves of the carbohydrates needed to run the energy factories of our body. We crave salt because we are deficient in minerals and have an imbalanced water organ system.

The Chinese pay attention to the five flavors of sweet, sour, pungent, bitter, and salty, as well as the five colors of black, white, green, yellow, and red. Each flavor and color corresponds to each of the five organ systems. By eating a diet that is balanced with the five flavors and five colors, the organ systems buzz harmoniously. Cravings are not an obstacle in a body that is nourished, balanced and cleansed.

# Chapter Six

✿

# Your Food

*"If we eat wrongly, No doctor can cure us; if we eat rightly, No doctor is needed."*

—Victor G. Rocine (1930)

My goal is to enlighten and teach the why and how of lifestyle changes. I teach the highest level of eating and I am not attached to whether a student chooses to eat a completely raw diet, or just 30% raw. Even the smallest steps this year will propel you to make bigger steps next year. It took years for me to be where I am at today. When I was an undergraduate student, I ate fast food and a lot of pizza. I was a huge eater when I was in my twenties. I would out-eat any guy in college. I could eat whole pies and pizzas in one sitting. I was never overweight, possibly because I had always worked out very hard. However, I certainly wasn't lean.

At the start of medical school, my diet consisted mainly of white bread sandwiches and cereal with cow's milk. During and after medical school, I removed meat, wheat and dairy from my diet. Although I felt better, the leap into vitality didn't come until I stopped cooking my food.

I had always suffered from chronic fatigue and intestinal problems, even with vegetarianism. With the huge amount of food I was eating, I wasn't having regular bowel movements. I slept 10 to 12 hours a day and was often lightheaded, especially during the premenstrual week. My lower abdomen was constantly distended; at times I looked like I was six months pregnant. I had moderate acne that started in my twenties. Both the bloating and acne got more severe during premenstrual time. As a naturopathic student, I was clueless about what might be wrong with me.

Throughout naturopathic school, I took herbs, glandulars, vitamins, ate like my peers, removed dairy from my diet—but none of these changes affected my state of health.

When I finally learned more about the body systems and their inner dynamics; when I finally realized I hadn't been feeding them the nutrients they needed in order to allow my body to first heal itself, my health started to turn around. I've now come to a place where I am no longer searching! I have found the answer to optimal health and higher mind. Today I am 15 pounds lighter than I used to be, and I'm stronger and much leaner. The biggest benefit

I've gained from eating mostly raw is the increased stamina and mental energy. I have never experienced momentum like I do now; the more raw my diet is, the better I feel and the less sleep I need. I would always envy people who were early risers. I could never seem to get up before 9:00 a.m.; it was a painful process. I always felt incredibly sluggish and dizzy. Now I bounce out of bed as early as 6:00 a.m., filled with energy and ready to meet the world head-on!

Before incorporating a somewhat raw diet, I was vegetarian for eight months. It wasn't until I started eating concentrated herbal foods that my body began the healing process by cleansing. Due to the amount of plant nutrition that was going into my body, my ravenous hunger decreased and I started eating less. I'm sure my exhausted digestive system was ecstatic about this, since it no longer had to work so hard. Vegetables began to taste so good, I found myself craving them. With more education, I started eating primarily raw fruits and vegetables, nuts and seeds. By the second day of eating completely raw, I could feel the difference. I lost 10 pounds in the first two weeks of eating raw. My bowels finally got the energy to release much of the stored toxic water and wastes from the huge meals I'd eaten years ago.

The undigested food products in an overworked bowel are absorbed into the intestinal lining for later elimination, when or if the body ever gets around to it. That's why the intestinal lining of some people can be up to 12 inches thick versus the normal 2 inches. Recall that the haustras in the colon allow for considerable expansion. My incredible distention was due to an expanded air- and water- filled colon. I know my colon was twisted in the upper and lower left quadrants where the colon makes its turns. After reading Dr. Bernard Jensen's book on colon health, I put the pieces of the puzzle together. As the feces accumulate in the colon, the muscles will contract to eliminate this waste. However, because of dehydration and poor energy, the contractions are ineffective. The combination of voluntary and involuntary straining to eliminate this waste over a long period of time leads to twisting of certain areas of the colon. The ileocecal valve in the lower right quadrant of the abdomen is often stuck, which can lead to constipation. The lower left quadrant where the sigmoid colon is located, gets the worst treatment. It balloons and twists, suffering from the massive amounts of old food waste that it cannot release.

A pure diet in combination with yoga and meditation has helped my colon to correct its deformations. Although the stomach and small intestine are quick to heal, the colon demands more time and care for it to recover from all of its injuries. So I will mention it again; patience is truly a virtue when choosing not to treat the symptoms, but instead to allow the body to bring itself into balance. Alternative modern day practitioners tend to prescribe short term liver and colon cleanses. In naturopathic medical school, this was the method for dealing with toxicity. However, the forceful cleanses never worked, not for myself or anyone I witnessed who was treated with a short term liver cleanse. I like to use the following analogy to explain a short term liver cleanse, which utilizes medicinal herbs and isolated fiber products.

You own a house and have housecleaners there every day to keep the house clean. They need certain tools in order to do their job. The housemaids also need energy in the form of nourishment and water. Let's say you starve them for a year and give them just one glass of water a day. You also don't give them any supplies, such as brooms or rags. At the same time, garbage is dumped into the house every day. Day after day the hungry, thirsty housemaids do the best they can to clean the house so that you can at least move around. They scavenge around looking for supplies to aid them in their cleaning. One morning you decide you're sick of living in filth because it's affecting your quality of life. So you pump the exhausted housecleaners full of stimulants and work them for 10 days straight, still without rest or nourishment. At the end of the 10 days they are completely exhausted and sick.

What are the stimulants I'm referring to? Anything that is isolated stimulates one or more organ systems of the body. Because the substances are not whole food and are synthetic concoctions, they are difficult to absorb. For the body to make use of these products, the liver, adrenal glands and immune system must all work together to use and eliminate these substances. Some of the cleansing products include isolate fiber products, medicinal herbs, isolate vitamins, minerals and digestive enzymes.

You are born with cleansing organs for your internal house. These precious organs need food and water to do their jobs properly, just like you need food and water to do your work each day. If given live nourishment and water, the eliminative organs clean house every single day to the best of their ability. As long as the burden is not too great they can do a magnificent job.

How do you treat your cleansing organs? Do you consume devitalized junk food and drink little or no water? This is the usual American lifestyle. The most reliable sign for liver and intestinal toxicity is fatigue. No wonder I was sleeping 12 hours a day! Vicarious elimination of toxins must take place in a weakened body in order to survive. This is done through sweat, skin outbreaks, mucus and emotions.

It is apparent to me that there is a difference between life and death. When a plant is fried, boiled, baked or steamed, it is dead. What separates a dead organism from a live one? They both have their anatomy and structures in place immediately after death; they appear to be the same.

Electricity, *Qi*, life force, Prana, whatever you want to call it, must be present to call something alive. Dr. Wayne Dyer is a member of the World Hunger Council. He tells of the organization's effort to create chemically manufactured wheat. In the lab, the creation looked exactly like the real deal. However, when planted in the ground the synthetic wheat didn't grow. What was missing? *Any artificial product lacks intelligence.* Intelligence is part of the magical essence, or life force of any natural product

In his book, *Fit for Life*, Harvey Diamond speaks of living foods as having "a body of light"; this has been proven through German research. He described living food as having "sophisticated cellular structures which incorporate spin-ahead and spin-reverse electrons that have aligned to produce pure light." A dense electron body (which he called a "light body") surrounds all living foods.

Humans have an energy body as well, called the *aura*. Every living thing is made up of atoms that are in constant motion. These atoms are made up of electrons, protons, and neutrons; we are dynamic, ever-changing beings. When we consume light bodies, we are recharged. When we consume a carcass or something that has had the life irradiated out of it, we are "zapped"; energy is taken from us.

Essence, as the Chinese call it, takes its form as enzymes. These biochemical complexes are the workers of the body, performing 2.5 million activities per minute. Enzymes consist of protein carriers charged with energy factors just as a battery consists of metallic plates charged with electrical energy. The human body has an estimated 50,000 enzymes.

These workers depend on coenzymes to function. The vitamins and minerals, which play the role of coenzymes, are analogous to the worker's tools. If you had a carpenter come over to fix your porch, would you tell him to leave his tools at home? If you boiled him first, do you think he could do any work? The answer makes sense to us in the outer world, but for some reason, unlike the Chinese, we cannot seem to accept the fact that the universe still continues to unfold in the dark stillness of the body.

Dr. Edward Howell, M.D., the world authority on enzymes, tells us of two kinds of enzymes, metabolic and digestive. Metabolic enzymes perform all the biochemical functions of the body. They depend on nutrients from the food to carry out their activities. The entire immune system runs its armies on metabolic enzymes. These workers also run the detoxification pathways of all the cells, manufacture all of our hormones and run our nervous system. They break down, clean up, and build anew. Enzymes also construct genetic material, and the genes in turn direct enzymatic activity in building proteins.

Digestive enzymes are the second type. They live in your digestive tract and their purpose is to break down the protein, fats, and carbohydrates into amino acids, fatty acids and glucose, respectively.

Dr. Howell compared our enzyme supply with that of a bank account full of money. The Chinese write that we are born with prenatal essence from the heavens and we acquire postnatal essence from our food. When we eat lifeless food we deplete our prenatal essence. In other words, if we withdraw more money from our God-given bank account than we deposit, we age quickly and degenerate before our time.

How about vitamins and minerals? Are they alive or are they just chemistries that can be manufactured in a lab? Vitamins are "accessory food substances" that are used in the assimilation of food and in directing minerals and enzymes. Dr. Bernard Jensen describes vitamins as "biological complexes, bundles of enzymes and trace minerals, biological wheels within wheels within wheels."

The first vitamin that was discovered and later synthetically made was vitamin A. If isolated from its counterparts and taken into the body, a synthetic vitamin such as vitamin A can be toxic if you consume too much. However when taken in its natural form, such as the beta-carotene in a carrot, it is never toxic, even if you juice 20 carrots. In medical school, we memorized the toxicity levels of isolate vitamins and minerals just as we memorized the toxicity levels of pharmaceutical drugs and medicinal herbs.

Synthetic vitamins are produced as the result of experiments performed on whole food. Vitamins were discovered in the early 1900s when certain foods were found to cure extreme vitamin deficiencies such as scurvy, beri beri, and pellagra. Cheap isolate vitamins and minerals were manufactured so that people could afford to get their vitamin needs met. Those extreme deficiency diseases no longer exist in this country, since almost everyone can afford to buy enough food. In actuality, the synthetics were never proven to cure any of the above mentioned diseases; only a food that was high in the needed vitamin cured scurvy, pellagra or beri beri.

Vitamin research is based on laboratory experiments in which a lab rat is deprived of one specific vitamin and all other variables are fixed. Since when do we live in a lab where there are no variables? If there is one thing we can count on in this world it is change, externally and internally. The environment in which we live is constantly changing and so are our bodies. Basic nutritional biochemistry tells us that if we are deficient in one vitamin, we are deficient in many more. The nutrients in our body are interdependent, so there is no such thing as being deficient in just one nutrient.

Vitamin C has received a lot of attention from the scientific community. Vitamin C was discovered in 1937 by Dr. Albert Szent Giorgi. Even though he won the Nobel Prize for his work, Giorgi stated that he could never cure scurvy with the lab reproduction of vitamin C, ascorbic acid. However, he could always rely on the "impure" batch of vitamin C that came from food. So he went back to the lab and discovered the rutin factor of the C complex that exists more in buckwheat than in citrus fruit.

Ascorbic acid is the synthetic form of vitamin C. Vitamin C as it exists in a lemon consists of a family of factors that includes copper, factor P, rutin factor, flavenoids, and the enzyme tyrosinase. Surrounding this gift of healing properties are the ascorbic acid rings. These rings revolve around the gift, fighting off free radicals to protect the delicate and valuable vitamin C package. Supplement manufacturers have extracted the ascorbic acid rings and then reproduced something that resembles it. It's like robbing a bank, taking the guards (ascorbic acid rings) and leaving the money (vitamin C package). And what is ascorbic acid made of? Corn syrup and volatile acids.

Dean Black, Ph.D., wrote a book about the context in which we live. Contextual healing, resembling the nature cure approach and traditional Chinese philosophy, was formerly more common than our current medical model. Contextual healers such as Hippocrates and the traditional Chinese doctors believe it is the context in which we live and how well we adapt to our context that determines our health. Some of the "context parameters" that we can adjust include: the food we eat, the air we breathe, the news we hear, the water we drink, the music we listen to, the books we read, how forgiving we are, how much we exercise, how much we rest, etc.

Following is a good analogy that uses this contextual idea. Your roommate buys an aquarium with some fish in it. On the first day, the water is clear and the fish are active. Night after night your roommate feeds the fish dinner leftovers of pizza, frozen dinners and some apple pie. Day after day, he neglects to change the water. By Friday, the water is turbid and you notice the fish are barely moving. You alert your friend and he declares, "Oh I know what they need, they need fish medicine from the doctor!" People usually laugh and say how ludicrous that is. It's obvious that if we change the water and feed the fish what it needs, they will thrive. Unfortunately we can get clear on something when it's on the outside or when it's not about us directly, but we struggle with clarity "on the inside"!

Our body cells are analogous to the fish suspended in an aquarium of interstitial fluid. We feed them garbage, never clean out the water and then give them cell medicine from the doctor when they don't work right. It's all too apparent that this method doesn't work. Like Pasteur said himself, "The terrain is everything, the germ is nothing."

I wholeheartedly believe that the research claiming the health benefits of isolate vitamins, minerals, and drugs has no validity. I learned this the painful way by climbing out of the muck and looking at my results. The results were obvious; I was in very poor health and had cabinets full of pharmaceutical grade supplements and medicinal herbs.

Let's revisit the discussion on enzymes and their coenzymes. Remember that the enzyme or worker needs his tools, which correlate to the vitamin and/or mineral associated with that enzyme. When you take a bottle of vitamins, you are ingesting a bunch of tools that have little use in the body. In fact, because of their poor absorption, their byproducts become toxic to the body. Nutritional scientists around the world confirm that at best you can absorb 10% of a synthetic nutrient.

First: how much did the body have to work in order to absorb 10% of that vitamin? It certainly had to complex the isolate with the rest of the components to make it whole again. This process stimulates the adrenal glands and burdens the liver.

Second: where does the other 90% go? The unabsorbed portion of the vitamin becomes another toxin the body must neutralize and eliminate. I've noticed that people who have taken a lot of supplements and switch to a nutrient-dense live food diet will cleanse considerably. It's not surprising, since they have years of chemical residue to get rid of.

How about the "natural" vitamins that are derived from food? Certainly they may have come from food, but before the extracted vitamins were put into capsules, the food went through heat, distillation, solvents and chemical treatment. The vitamin, through the process of extraction, was separated from its family of trace minerals and enzymes that were in the original food.

We have over 75 trillion cells that have individual needs. Do we really want to play chemist for each of those cells? Taking too much of one vitamin causes a deficiency in another vitamin and/or mineral. For example, women are told to take 1500 mg of calcium daily, and the body only needs 150 mg per day. Taking too much calcium lowers phosphorus, magnesium, and sodium levels. When the mineral ratios are thrown out of balance, you could take 5,000 mg of calcium daily for your bones and it wouldn't make a bit of difference. The only effect it would have on your body is the formation of kidney stones and bone spurs. Acidic diets and malabsorption are the two causes of rampant osteoporosis in this country. Minerals are alkaline and are used in the body as buffers. In an acidic environment, in order to keep you alive and balance the pH of your blood, the body is forced to leech the alkaline minerals from the bones, hair and teeth. Numerous studies have shown that calcium supplements are useless, and that eliminating the acidifying foods such as protein and dairy will allow your body to rebuild the bones. You may even stop losing your hair and have healthier teeth.

Taking too much zinc and niacin can lower copper. Mega-doses of vitamin C lower B12. Many people are told to take B vitamins, especially vegetarians. Little do they know that synthetic vitamin B comes from coal tar and B12 comes from activated sewage sludge. When isolated, vitamin B12 is highly mutable, making it useless to the body. It is a common belief that the only way to get B12 is from animal meat. It's true that animals produce significantly more B12 than plants. Accordingly, the human body makes its own B12 through the activity of microbial life. Under the tongue, between the teeth, through the bile and in our intestines, B12 is produced in sufficient amounts.

Various medical sources agree that we need between .25-.5 micrograms per day of B12. This is 250 to 500 times less than the microgram tablets offered by the supplement companies. These numbers show us the extraordinary amount of the synthetic form that is never absorbed by the body. Vegetarians need not worry about their B12, since they have been shown to absorb a much higher percentage of B12 than a meat-eater. This is one example of how the body adapts to the context of diet.

I had a patient who relied on weekly B12 shots from her doctor because part of her intestines had been removed. She had trouble holding on to things and would black out. These symptoms are evident in a B12 deficiency. When she came to me, she discontinued the B12 shots and conformed to the nutrient dense herbal food diet. I did not give her any vitamins. She stopped dropping things and blacking out. Her body now had enough raw materials to manufacture the B12 in the secondary places of the body. This is one case of many that revealed to me the power of the human body, when given what it needs to rebalance itself.

Plants have hundreds of thousands of nutrient substances that have not yet been identified. No one knows how many nutritive constituents there are in an orange. Beta-carotene is just one of over 600 substances classified as carotenoids, which are found in yellow and orange fruits and vegetables. When taking a synthetic beta-carotene, the cell receptor sites for carotenoids are flooded with this one isolate, which excludes the use of all of the other carotenoids needed by the body. A study of 30,000 Finnish subjects published in the *New England Journal of Medicine* reported that the subjects who received synthetic B-carotene had an increased level of heart attacks, strokes and lung cancer, compared to those who received the placebo. I thought B-carotene was supposed to help with cardiovascular disease.

Vitamin A is associated with many other components including retinols, retinoids, retinal, carotenes, fatty acids, vitamin C, E, B, D, enzymes and minerals. Taking the isolate vitamin A depletes the body of all these other components, while exposing the cells to large amounts of a strong chemical.

The discoverer of thiamin and the man who came up with the word vitamin, Dr. Casimir Funk, said the following about synthetics: "Synthetic vitamins are highly inferior to vitamins from natural sources; also the synthetic product is well known to be far more toxic." In his book, *Superior Nutrition*, Herbert Shelton wrote: "Man's ills are not to be remedied by fragments, but by proper use of all of the related elements of his basic needs in organic unity." *Suum Cuique tributio*—give to each its own. The body desires food substances that are similar to the essence of its tissues.

Only a few plant chemicals, such as flavenoids, mucilages, phenols, glycosides, catechins, bitters, saponins, coumarins, and alkaloids, have been discovered. These plant chemicals, called phytonutrients, offer extraordinary benefits to the body, and we have yet to discover the full range of their benefits. What we do know is that they offer potent antioxidant and cancer fighting properties, increase metabolism, facilitate digestion and assimilation, catalyze detoxification of toxins, reduce inflammation, and increase organ adaptability. These are just a few of the functions these miracle substances perform in the body.

The word medicine in Chinese means "plants to enjoy." Uncooked, plants are the only means by which we obtain live enzymes, vitamins, minerals, and thousands of phytonutrients, most of which have not yet been discovered. Most vitamins lose their potency at about 212 degrees.

Enzymes are fragile, affected by light, heat, and pressure. They are deactivated at temperatures exceeding 118 degrees.

Proteins have a specific chemical shape that makes it possible for a digestive enzyme to lock and key it. When cooked, the protein chains lose their characteristic shapes and become denatured or no longer recognizable to our protein digesting enzymes. It's like changing the lock on your door and still using the old key. As a result, undigested proteins in the body expose us to harmful byproducts such as ammonia, which behaves like chemicals that cause or promote cancer.

Since the 1930s, studies have reported a phenomenon known as leukocytosis in response to cooked food. Leukocytosis is defined as an increase in white blood cells, which essentially means the immune system is stimulated by the cooked food. Proteins that never got disassembled into amino acids in the small intestine escape into the blood. In response to the presence of large proteins in the blood, antibodies attack the protein, forming an antibody-antigen complex. The immune system becomes chronically hyperactive in response to the regular onslaught of foreign proteins in the blood. This immune response can explain most allergies, autoimmune diseases, fibromyalgia, chronic arthritis, chronic fatigue, and most of the immunodeficiency diseases.

We absorb uncooked protein much better than cooked protein. It is not necessary to consume 75 to 100 grams of daily protein as suggested by commercial interests. When taken in the unaltered form, our digestive enzymes are able to extract from the protein the amino acids that we need. Amino acids themselves are made up of vibrating atoms. When these are heated, the vibration is deadened, making the amino acids useless. These dead bodies congest our tissues and contribute to the acidic waste that spawns disease.

Processed food creates mutagens in the body that can alter the DNA. Weston Price, D.D.S., published his paramount studies on world nutrition in 1939 in *Nutrition and Physical Degeneration.* He studied the effects of adulterated foods on indigenous societies and found that when the parents ate the foods of commerce, they passed along inferior genetic traits to the next generation. In the conclusion of his book, Dr. Price wrote, "Even heredity with all its complicated nature, while in a sense immortal is itself purely physical and composed of units of proteins, minerals and vitamins called genes . . ." Have you noticed that we are forever hearing from the media about yet another new genetic phenomenon? Recently I met a woman whose family supposedly has a gene that will cause stomach cancer and the recommendation is to remove the stomach. To my dismay, some of her family members have had their stomachs removed even when no disease was present.

Another effect of cooked or processed food is the softening of food fibers, which can hamper intestinal mobility.

Demagnetized fibers leave behind a slimy coating. Cooked carbohydrates become caramalized and dextrinized, which causes weight gain.

Raw foods are digested easily in 24 to 36 hours as opposed to 48 to100 hours for cooked food. Eating raw foods not only provides a substantial amount of nutrients over cooked foods; their metabolism also does not leave any toxic residue or other byproducts.

Previously I mentioned the five flavors and colors of foods that indicate their benefits to the body. Nature uses taste as an offering of balance to the body. *Sweet* foods are light, curb hunger and nourish the body. Natural sugars increase tissue mass, since glucose is the main fuel for all body processes. Sweet flavored foods act upon the stomach, spleen and pancreas. Most fruits, especially dates and figs, are sweet.

*Salty* foods are heavier. Sodium follows water so that salt flavored foods affect water movement in the body. Sodium is important for softening tissues such as ligaments and tendons. All vegetables contain natural sodium.

*Pungent* foods are spicy and heating to the body. Cayenne and ginger are well known for their positive effect on blood circulation. They act on the lungs and large intestine and help to open things up and clear mucus.

*Bitter* foods act on the heart and small intestine. They are cooling, light and dry. Green leafy vegetables such as endive, escarole, and watercress have this quality.

*Sour* foods such as lemons affect the liver and gall bladder. They improve digestion and aid in detoxification.

A great dressing that will satisfy all five tastes is made with Bragg Liquid Aminos, lemon juice and cold pressed olive oil or some other therapeutic oil such as flax oil or Udo's oil. For a more salty flavor, you can use Gomasio. Gomasio is made with sesame seeds and sea salt. The ratio is 8 parts seeds to one part sea salt. You can find Gomasio on the internet or in a health food store. You can find Udo's oil in the refrigerator in most health food stores. Udo's oil is my favorite; it has a mixture of plant oils that provide the omega 3, 6, and 9 fatty acids. It is better to eat the oils from plants rather than the fish oil products that are being marketed, and it is better to eat the whole fish for dinner if you want some of those oils in your body.

Whenever someone asks what they should eat, my answer is anything that grows out of the dirt. Eating a wide variety of fruits and vegetables, mostly seasonal, is the finest way to eat. Occasional grains are acceptable as a building food. Quinoa is a grain that has 5g of protein per serving and lots of fiber. I like it as a background food for my salads. Other grains that are similar to quinoa are amaranth and millet. Remember to eat grains only occasionally.

Legumes are high in potassium and phosphorus. Chard, kale and broccoli are very high in calcium. Raw nuts and seeds are good sources of protein. Cabbage is high in vitamin C and A, and is cleansing to the body. Dandelion greens, beets, garlic, and lemons are known for their benefits to the liver. Unrefined nuts, seeds, and grains are high in silicon. The trace mineral silicon is necessary for brain function and also benefits the alimentary tract and lungs.

Celery, cabbage and strawberries are good sources of sodium. Organic sodium is necessary for the sodium potassium pump to run and is one of the main ions in your extracellular fluid. Sodium benefits the ligaments and joints. Sodium also neutralizes acids and works with chlorine to help cleanse the body.

The good fats are found in raw nuts and seeds, coconut, cold pressed olive oil, or Udo's oil and avocados. As you can see, no one vegetable, fruit or grain will meet all of your nutritional needs. By eating a wide variety of fresh fruits and vegetables you will get your entire vitamin, mineral, and protein needs met. Making sure they are alive and not cooked or processed will ensure that you are depositing ample enzymes into your bank account.

Juicing your fruits and vegetables is effective for concentrating the nutrients, which is necessary these days due to the innate nutritional deficiencies in the American grown plants.

Fluids deserve a special mention as their importance cannot be emphasized enough. What else is there to say, except drink, drink, drink! Whether you're thirsty or not, drink. You should be urinating once every hour to an hour-and-a- half. Keep in mind that your body is mostly fluid. Toxins are flushed out by liquids, joints are lubricated by fluid, enzymes need fluid, your blood needs fluid, and your intestines need fluid. Unless you want to be constructed of stiff, dry tissues with stuck-on grease, I recommend you drink 4 to 5 quarts of water every day.

Your plasma is similar to ocean water. It contains electrolytes, minerals and salts. Therefore, I add plant food to my water. Your body would prefer fresh water from a river bed instead of dead water from a plastic bottle. You will definitely feel the difference when you enliven your water with plant food. If you live in the desert, drinking 4 to 5 quarts in the winter and 5 to 7 quarts in the summer is strongly recommended. Even if you live in Virginia you need to drink at least 4 quarts per day. Would you ever run your car without oil? Drink!

# Chapter Seven

꘏꘏꘏

# Your Mind

*There is a Power that will light your way to health, happiness, peace, and success, if you will but turn toward that Light.*

— Paramahansa Yogananda

As mentioned before, eastern philosophy emphasizes the importance of balanced emotions. Because each organ system bears a certain energetic vibration, our feelings carry a great deal of power as they flow through the body.

There's a lot of buzz these days about the integration of mind and feelings being the secret to success. I do believe this to be true. I have found personally that when I think, feel and do the same thing, I reach success in a particular endeavor. It is when I think one thing, feel another and do something entirely different that my desired result fails to come to fruition.

Alignment is important because a thought causes us to feel a certain way, which in turn motivates us to take action or make a decision. Usually actions are initiated by having some feeling or emotional response to something. The feeling would not have occurred if the thought hadn't been there first. Many teachers of ancient wisdom as well as today's motivational leaders claim that "to think is to create." I believe this idea has some validity. The sequence for manifesting results is: thought-feeling-action-result.

Several questions arise as to how we can align ourselves. Equally important is knowing when we are out of alignment. It is impossible to keep track of the all the thoughts that go through our heads, most of them coming from the subconscious mind. Psychologists have proven that you produce between 50,000 and 75,000 thoughts a day and eighty percent of these thoughts are negative. Therefore, by age forty you have had 730,000,000 (730 million) thoughts. If eighty percent of your thoughts are negative, then the slate of your mind is layered with 584,000,000 negative thoughts. This means even if you were to do 500 positive affirmations a day, trying to reprogram your mind to be positive, your mind would be sub-vocalizing 40,000 negative thoughts to the contrary.

Many people do positive affirmations every day; I used to do this. They definitely have their place but are not the end-all to changing one's life. If you want love in your life but your mind is filled with failed relationship thoughts, it will not matter if you say "love is grand" a thousand times or more, because the affirmation lacks feeling. In contrast, the negative thoughts surrounding your past failed relationships carry a strong emotional charge. This charge is so powerful it can even alter the cells of your physical body. The negative charge goes out to the world and attracts what you don't want: another failed relationship. So we're back to where we started—which is to ask, where do we start?

Since our thoughts initiate our feelings, monitoring our thoughts could be the answer to changing how we feel. Then if we feel differently, we would make different choices, leading to different results. However, according to the numbers previously quoted, it is humanly impossible to keep track of our thoughts!

The best way to gauge how aligned you are, is to look at your results. I heard this saying years ago and hold it close to my heart because it is the only way I can keep track of myself: "Results, often harsh always fair." Only by measuring your results in life can you see what your subconscious is up to. What are your results? Meaning, how much money do you have in the bank? Do you or your boss have control over your time? Do you have strong intimate relationships in your life? How is your health?

From your subconscious mind flood thousands of unruly thoughts, each attached to their feeling vibrations. When averaged together, these thoughts will cause you to make a decision or take a particular action. This activity in turn leads to a particular result.

By looking at your results *without judgment*, you can trace backwards to the action, feeling and original thought that initiated this process. You can go back even further by tracing the underlying thought to some past experience that left a mark in your subconscious. By releasing your judgment of that experience, perhaps you can neutralize the emotional charge on that thought. As long as the thought does not carry an emotional charge, it will not create an action. So you can be assured that just by looking at your results and the actions you took to achieve those results, you will be guided to the emotionally charged thoughts. This tracking procedure has given me a way to "watch" my subconscious mind. Of course it is impossible as a human to be completely aware of the depths of one's mind, but at least this process gives me a way of changing many areas of my life. It has been proven to be very effective, since I have made a number of dramatic changes within an extremely short period of time! Today, I have the freedom of managing my own time, a loving intimate relationship, dear friends and a healthy body.

As always, I have ongoing work to do on myself to preserve my inner peace and not allow it to be curtailed by circumstances. This has been challenging for me, but the outcome will certainly be worth the effort. I firmly believe that when you have achieved unshakable inner peace, you will have everything you want, whether you are materially rich or not.

My definition of success is inner peace and inner joy. If I have both of these, it doesn't matter if I'm sitting in a prison cell or in the finest home in the world.

Recently I stayed at an upscale resort for a weekend, just to unwind. During that time I witnessed people arguing, drinking, smoking and indulging in other numbing activities such as overeating and overworking. In the past year I have been meditating and doing yoga on a daily basis. Because of the change in my inner world, I have become sensitive to the vibrations of those who are not peaceful on the inside. It took me a full 24 hours to feel like myself again after leaving that resort; in fact, I checked out early! The people staying there no doubt were materially wealthy but I felt they were impoverished spiritually and emotionally.

All the money in the world means nothing to me without my sense of inner joy and calmness. If I had to choose between material and spiritual wealth, I would choose to be wealthy as a soul rather than as a body. Don't you know that you will be leaving this shell behind in just a few years?

The good news is, we don't have to choose. I've brought this matter of material versus spiritual wealth to your attention so that when you define what success means to you, you'll be honest with yourself. What makes you happy, really? I mean really. You want to get so real with yourself right now that you're brought to tears. In purifying the body, mucus comes out; in purifying the soul, tears come forth.

Once you discover through conscious awareness how you operate, then you can become the captain of your ship. Who is the *you* that I'm referring to? The you that needs to be in charge of your life is your higher self.

If you recall, your spirit is divided into prenatal and postnatal essences. Your prenatal essence is born of the cosmos and can be referred to as the super-conscious mind. Your postnatal essence is earth-bound and can be referred to as the ego or conscious mind.

Your subconscious mind dwells between the two; I believe it contains parts of both the super-conscious and conscious minds. Your conscious mind filters sensory stimuli and perceptions, feeding most of them into your subconscious mind. This part is definitely the egoistic aspect. Yet, your dreams and memories of past life experiences that reside in your subconscious mind will travel through time and space into other dimensions, likened to your super-conscious mind.

Your super-conscious mind is your individualized spirit or soul. This is the *yin* aspect, and the ego is the *yang* aspect.

*Yin* is quiet, in the dark, and flowing. *Yang* is loud, in the light, and forceful. *Yin* is female; *yang* is male. If you want to personalize these two beings within you, then you can say that you have a male side and a female side. Henceforth, I will be referring to your higher self in the feminine gender and your ego in the male gender.

Personalizing the different aspects of my being helped me a great deal. I now had a way to parent myself so that when I say I want something, I actually take the correct steps to achieve it. Self-sabotage is the result of not being aligned. Saying one thing and doing another is the biggest self-sabotage I can think of. By not being in integrity with yourself, you are not in integrity with others.

Lack of integrity, I believe is the culprit behind low self-esteem. Lack of integrity and low self-esteem create a positive feedback cycle. When you don't do what you say you're going to do, you take a chip out of your self-esteem. When your self-esteem is low, you follow through even less with your commitments.

This is where compassion comes in. When you notice you're late all the time or fail to fulfill the commitments you make to yourself and others, you must realize that you have a poor self-image. If you take steps to nourish yourself physically, mentally, and spiritually you can break this painful cycle. For example, keeping to one's diet and exercise plan requires that you practice integrity. Once you fall off the wagon one time, be aware that your self-esteem takes a hit. However, if you control your thoughts, you can use willpower to get yourself back on track.

This brings me to my next important point, willpower. With willpower you have the potential to override the darkness of your subconscious mind and literally change the patterns of your behavior. Willpower is exercised when you do something you don't feel like doing and yet you know it is in your higher interest. For the moment, you are accepting that you are out of alignment and you are going to act without the initiating feeling.

Earlier, we were talking about how thought begets feeling and feeling begets action, which leads to a particular result. Now, you will go backwards by doing the action which will change how you feel, which will then lead to positive thoughts about yourself.

Exercise and diet are great opportunities for practicing willpower. Success in following a routine we've created for ourselves can dramatically change our self-esteem. When you feel good about yourself, you are no longer paralyzed by fear. You make the phone calls you need to make; you approach people with your ideas; you start writing, painting and hoping again, without the fear of failure.

I'm sure all of us know of someone in our lives or we've read about someone who was overweight. After they lost that extra weight, their life changed radically. Even their personality may have changed. Perhaps they became more outgoing and engaged more intimately with others; perhaps they became more assertive in their career. They now make more money, have better relationships, etc. All of this happened because they disciplined themselves to eat better and exercise on a consistent and regular basis. I've heard many stories of cancer survivors who are healthier than they've ever been in their life and have completely changed their attitudes, relationships and careers.

I particularly remember my mentor, Colleen, telling us about the chain of life with its different links: emotional, mental, spiritual, and physical. When I didn't have my health, I did tons of affirmations and tried to "think" myself to health. However, at the time I didn't know what to eat, so the affirmations weren't enough. Once I learned about the Chinese herbal foods and the benefits of raw foods, I got my health back. With renewed energy, all the different areas of my life started to change rapidly. I had the willpower; I just didn't have the tools. You may have the tools, but perhaps you don't have a strong will.

Your willpower is a mental muscle that you may not have exercised before. Without willpower, you are operating completely by autopilot, following your whims and not looking at the long term consequences. Unfortunately, the law of cause and effect never ceases to rest and before long you will feel the effect of your indulgences. There is always time to change one's mind, however. That's all it takes: an attitude adjustment by the power of your will.

Train the mind to be the servant of your soul. Most people are being ruled by their lower mind and have lost connection with their higher self. Daily introspection through meditation and yoga practices will bring your soul forth into your consciousness so you can start to feel the difference between lower and higher vibrations. Once you can experience the difference, you can use your discrimination to do only those things which transport you to higher states of consciousness. Merely recognizing how you feel when you think a negative thought or succumb to a bad habit will prompt you to strengthen your willpower to avoid those habits in the future.

I have recognized through difficult trials and the humility they brought me, that without God or a higher power, I am just a little person. This is not a religious statement, but I must be honest. We humans are not the doers. Without this cosmic power, we cease to breathe. You will learn this kind of humility through the trials of life; one day you will be brought to your knees in humility with the realization that you cannot do it alone. This day can be the best day of your life, if you choose to embrace the heavens and work with the universal laws rather than against them.

I have even learned to depend on God to give me the willpower to evolve my soul. I can't just drum up willpower;

it's not really mine to begin with. So I ask for God's will to be made manifest through me. The burden is much lighter and I am much more effective in making changes in my life when I don't allow my ego to get too involved in the process.

At this point I would like to discuss intention versus mechanism in relation to the three levels of knowing that were mentioned at the beginning of this book. These three concepts can really move you forward once you've decided where you want to go. All that's necessary is to follow your heart.

I want to stop here for a moment and define "heart." Following your heart does not mean to follow your emotions. By heart, I mean your soul or higher self that expresses through your feelings. We must learn to decipher between our feelings and our emotions. Emotions are passionate and volatile. Feelings are more stable and intuitive. It will take practice for you to get to know yourself in this way; be patient.

I want to review the three levels of knowing, as they are crucial in evaluating your progress. The first level of knowing is the way a student knows the answers to exam questions. At this level, the information is purely intellectual. In other words, no changes are made based on the learned information. When you take this academic knowledge out into the world and start practicing it, you will see if it is true for you.

This brings us to the second level of knowing. You've heard or read the information and now you believe it to be true. Does this mean you are practicing it in real life? Did you know that exercise and eating vegetables is good for you? Usually the answer is yes—yet many are not practicing the good habits of health. Hence, the information is still at the intellectual level. How many self-help books have you read that tell you some of the very same things I've written in this chapter? Why have you chosen to not put these ideals into practice? It could be because you still don't have the tools. Or it could be that you are not yet in enough pain to implement daily changes. The human is motivated by pleasure or pain. Nonetheless, the promise of pleasure or the feeling of pain must be great enough to move us to change our habits.

The third level of knowing is when you've heard or read the information, you believe it to be true, *and* you are practicing these ideas on a consistent basis. This level of knowing can be evidenced by one's results. By looking at the results in your life, you will know whether or not you are at the third level of knowing. As soon as you start exercising and eating right, you will be healthier. Good health is an outcome that reflects positive physical habits.

Once you start to practice self-control and do inward activities such as meditation and yoga, other positive changes will come about, such as greater prosperity and better relationships. These positive results will reflect to yourself and others that you must be practicing the universal truths. Finally, once you are inwardly joyful and peaceful regardless of the circumstances, then you have been practicing the highest ideals taught by the masters of ancient science.

There is no time better than right now to begin practicing those things you know to be true. Get up early tomorrow morning, sit still, and go within. Then exercise and eat a healthy light breakfast. Do it again the next day. Use your willpower until you can't breathe without practicing these good habits! If you feel mentally weak, get down on your knees and ask your Source for the will to make these changes.

Take responsibility for your life by knowing the difference between intention and mechanism. Intention is all that is needed to bring about the results you want. You can plan the logistics of a business for years or do research on a book for a decade, but that doesn't mean that just because you've taken these preliminary steps, a business will grow or a book will be written. At some point you need to start writing and at some point you need to start marketing your product! Without intention, you can be stuck your whole life in the mechanism of planning and discussing the how to's of making something happen.

Too often, we blame our circumstances for our lack of momentum. We literally get stuck in our own stories and excuses, as well as those of others. Free yourself from this prison that your mind has built out of laziness. You must be honest with yourself so you know where you stand. What is *really* stopping you from growing your business or finding true love? **Fear.**

We make the mechanism so important in our minds because we are scared to death of failure or rejection, or of just plain looking stupid. I've read many times about the countless mistakes that successful people have made on their climb upward. Of course they made huge mistakes, because they were taking huge risks! What's the point of playing it safe? Did you know that you have 100% chance of dying? So, whether you die broke or rich is beside the point. But did you live? Did you give of yourself when you thought you had nothing to give? Did you go after your goals each day as if it was your last?

Recognize that whatever your results, it is because you intended them to be that way, consciously or subconsciously. They just didn't happen to you. Even if you consciously did all that you could do to make that failed relationship successful, your subconscious mind sabotaged it. It may then become apparent to you that you must have a subconscious intention to experience a failed relationship. Further introspection may reveal feelings of low self-worth that keep attracting the wrong type of person for an intimate relationship, or for any type of relationship—friendship, professional, etc.

This means you must take responsibility for your subconscious as well as your conscious intentions, since they both produce the results in your life. In fact, I would guess that since most people don't use their willpower, the subconscious mind is basically living their life for them. Only by taking complete responsibility for your results, actions, feelings and thoughts, can you ever change these patterns.

You have chosen, with intention, to be where you are at today. As you start to make changes in your life, continually introspect by noticing your actions. If you are constantly late to work, then clearly it is your subconscious intention to be fired from that job. If you tell yourself that you are going to be nicer to your mate but you still blow up at them, then clearly it is your intention to not be in that relationship. It could be from feelings of unworthiness or your higher self prompting you to be alone or leave that job. You will need to do some serious introspection to figure it out.

I have noticed that when I secretly wished for a person or situation to move out of my life, something happened within a short period of time that accomplished that wish, without any action on my part. So the saying, "be careful what you wish for," definitely rings true for me. Also, as you become more aligned, so will your wishes become more powerful.

Whatever you put your *attention* to becomes your *intention*. If you pay more attention to how fat you are, then by matter of law, it is your intention to be fat. If you are always thinking about your bills, then it is your intention to always have bills.

*Focus on what you want, not on what you don't want.* By changing your attention, you change your intention. Instead of focusing on how fat you feel, focus on how good you are going to feel when you change your diet and start exercising. Instead of focusing on your debt, be creative in coming up with solutions to increase your cash flow.

All the good health and vitality is yours for the taking if you just open your mind's eye to the gifts that are waiting for you to accept. All the prosperity of the universe is yours, if you will just feel more abundant.

How can one feel abundant without having a lot of money? Doesn't that feel like a lie? Doing affirmations for abundance, without the feeling behind them, means that you are thinking one thing and feeling another; this will not produce any results. You cannot just *think* your way to financial freedom; you must *feel* it.

The best way to prompt the feeling of abundance is through gratitude. I don't care what your circumstances are; you do have something to be grateful for. Even if there is only one good thing in your life, then dwell on that one good thing. This will elevate your thought vibrations, which will go out to the world and bring back more thoughts of like vibrations. Once your internal vibration is increased, you will start attracting the people and things you need in order to change your circumstances. So if you are breathing, and especially if you have a home and some food, you have plenty to be grateful for.

Outreach is another thing you can do to feel abundant. Instead of wallowing in self-pity, reach out to those who are less fortunate than you. Give money, time and smiles to those who need a lift. I can't tell you how good I feel when I'm outwardly focused. These positive feelings created by your actions will go out to the world and bring back to you all the resources you need to change your unfavorable circumstances.

Make the effort to not think about what's wrong in your life. After all, your problems will be there whether you think about them or not. Fill your head with hopes, dreams, chants and prayers, and watch your life change, with no or little effort on your part. You will begin to receive wonderful ideas and blessings.

Finally, take care of your soul. It's the only thing you will be taking with you when you depart from this life. When you care for her, she will bring to you all that life can offer. Follow the light by going within and asking for help. Be courageous and don't take yourself so seriously. I would like to end with a quote from the immortal master, Paramahansa Yogananda:

*O Spirit, teach me to find the fountain of infinite power within myself, that I may drink of its soothing waters and quench the thirst of all my needs.*

# Appendix

In his book, *The Complete System of Healing*, Stephen Chang, M.D., states, "regular foods do not provide enough nutrients to maintain a continuous state of health and must be supplemented by stronger, herbal foods." He also said that when foods are broken down to isolated chemicals, their synergy is destroyed. The synergy of the whole is much more powerful than the isolated parts.

Most of us are aware that we are not getting the nutrients we need from supermarket food. Due to soil depletion, these fruits and vegetables offer little nutrients. In the 1930s the Senate Select Committee on Health reported that we couldn't fit enough fruits and vegetables in our stomach to get the amount of nutrients we need every day in order to maintain optimal health. Furthermore, if you need to reverse a disease process, then you require even more nutrients than a healthy person.

More people are juicing as a way to concentrate the nutrition from their food. I always recommend juicing; but remember, every fruit and vegetable has traces of residue and you are concentrating these toxic residues when you juice. I tell people to use a veggie wash to minimize the amount of chemicals in the juice.

I have mentioned Chinese Herbal Foods throughout the book. These are similar to juiced fruits and vegetables. However, they are heirloom plants and have been growing for thousands of years. In addition, the plants used in the formulas are researched to feed specific organs. Every organ of your body needs its own particular nutrients to function properly. The Chinese were diligent in studying the effects of certain plants on the body. Moreover, the herbal foods that I eat are free of chemical residue. The formulator, Dr. Chen, understands the importance of chemical free plants when eating them in concentrated form. The plants are soaked in herbal soups and dried. The Essence and *Qi* are left intact during the concentration and drying process. The consumer receives them packaged for convenience.

You will feel the difference with the first shake and tea you drink. I start everyone on the foundational foods, which are NuPlus, Quinary, Calli tea, and Fortune Delight; the latter are herbal beverages. I also include Sunny Dew, which contains stevia and feeds the adrenal glands and pancreas.

NuPlus and Quinary contain plants that nourish all the organ systems of the body. These two formulas are concentrated and together consist of a total of over 60 plants.

Most people would like to look younger, have more energy and heal themselves of chronic ailments. To accomplish this, we have to have enough fuel for the body to rebuild itself while performing necessary daily functions. This requires three servings each of NuPlus and Quinary every day. People who eat only two servings a day of these vital herbal foods may notice more energy at breakfast time and for a few hours, but only after they increase their consumption of NuPlus and Quinary to three meals per day do dramatic changes take place. This is because increased consumption of these valuable nutrients gives the body enough energy to cleanse itself.

Only by cleansing can the body regenerate. This means that in order to have a new body, the old must be cleansed out. In an earlier chapter, we discussed the seven priorities of the body. The sixth and seventh priorities of regeneration and a higher mind require three meals every day. In addition to the NuPlus and Quinary, eat fresh fruits and vegetables, raw nuts and seeds. And don't forget your essential oils!

To assist your eliminative organs, there's nothing better than the Calli tea and Fortune Delight. These two beverages contain plants that have an affinity for the liver, kidneys, and intestines. By waking up these sluggish organs, they start to unload years of morbid waste. Drinking two quarts of Calli and two quarts of Fortune Delight every day will not only hydrate and cleanse your cells; it will also facilitate a daily cleansing regime so you will not build up toxic waste again. By cleansing every day, you feel vibrant and have mental clarity as you go about your day.

It is important to note that these herbal foods do not heal diseases. They are simply the raw materials the body will use to heal itself. *They are foods, not medicine.* Thus, the responsibility is yours to heal your body. If you want to be well, the first step is to eat wholesome, nourishing foods such as the ones I've listed. The next step is to take a leadership role in all areas of your life.

If you are eating these wonderful foods and would like guidance, please visit my website at:

www.communityofhigherliving.com.

*. . .the whole body is fitted together perfectly, and each part in its own way helps the other parts, so that the whole body is healthy and growing and full of love.*

— Ephesians 4:16

# About the Author

Dr. Jane Hendricks received her doctorate in Naturopathic Medicine from Southwest College of Naturopathic Medicine in 2002. Naturopathic physicians are licensed in Arizona with the scope of primary care doctors. They are trained in pharmaceuticals, minor surgery, intravenous therapies, supplementation and nutrition, chiropractic, homeopathy, medicinal herbs, acupuncture and Chinese medicine. They can specialize in obstetrics, pediatrics, and geriatrics or be generalized as family doctors.

Dr. Hendricks believes in the use of food to facilitate the body's own healing processes. Because of her own chronic illness as a student, she kept searching for answers beyond the supplements and medicinal herbs, as these offered no resolution for her ailments. In 2003 she began eating Chinese Herbal Foods. Her body cleansed out the stagnant toxins which resulted in a complete healing of her imbalances, along with a vitality she had never felt before. Her Irritable Bowel Disease and chronic fatigue of 15 years resolved.

Shortly thereafter, she closed her medical practice to work full time teaching the power of these Chinese Herbal Foods. She holds weekly classes to instruct and empower her students to nourish themselves to health. Dr. Hendricks' website is _www.communityofhigherliving.com_.

# References

Arlin, Stephen, Fouad, Dini, Wolfe, David, *Nature's First Law: The Raw Food Diet*. San Diego, California: Maul Brothers Publishing, 1996.

Arlin, Stephen, *RawPower*. San Diego, California: Maul Brothers Publishing, 1998.

Black, Dean, PhD, *Inner Wisdom*. Springville, Utah: Tapestry Press, 1990.

Bragg, Paul and Patricia, *The Shocking Truth about Water*. Santa Barbara, California: Health Science.

Cousins, Gabriel, M.D., *Conscious Eating*. Patagonia, AZ: Essene Vision Books, 1992.

Deng Liangyue, Gan Yijun, He Shuhui, *Chinese Acupuncture and Moxibustion*. Beijing: Foreign Language Press, 1987.

Dalconzo, Joseph Hu, *Self-Mastery*. Renaissance Publishing, 2002.

Diamond, Harvey, *Fit For Life*. New York, New York: Kensington Books, 2000.

Dubos, Rene and Pines, Maya, *Health and Disease, Life Science Library*. New York: Time Life Books, 1965.

Haas, Elson M.D., *Staying Health with the Seasons*. Berkeley, California: Celestial Arts, 1981.

Issels, Josef M.D., *Cancer, A Second Opinion*. Garden City Park, New York: Avery Publishing Group, 1999.

Jensen, Bernard and Anderson, Mark, *Empty Harvest*. Garden City Park, New York: Avery Publishing Group, 1990.

Jensen, Bernard, *Foods That Heal*. Garden City Park, New York: Avery Publishing Group, 1988.

Jensen, Bernard D.C., *Tissue Cleansing Through Bowel Management*. Escondido, California: Bernard Jensen Enterprises, 1981.

Kaptchuk, Ted O.M.D., *The Web That Has No Weaver*. Chicago, Illinois: Congdon & Weed, Inc., 1983.

Lindlahr, Henry M.D., *Philosophy of Natural Therapeutics*. England: C.W. Daniel Company Limited, 1975.

Mars, Brigitte, *Rawsome*. North Bergen, NJ: Basic Health Publications, Inc., 2004.

Mills, Simon and Bone, Kerry, *Principles and Practice of Phytotherapy*. Churchill Livingston, 2000.

O'Shea, Tim, *Sanctity of Human Blood*. San Jose, California: New West, 2001.

O'Shea, Tim, *Whole Food Vitamins: Ascorbic Acid Is Not Vitamin C.*

Pfeiffer, John, *The Cell, Life Science Library*. New York: Time Life Books, 1964.

Reid, Daniel, *The Complete Book of Chinese Health & Healing*. New York: Barnes & Noble Books, 1998.

Robbins, Joel, *The Food Revolution*. Berkeley, California: Conari Press, 2001.

Sebrell, William Jr. and Haggerty, James, *Food and Nutrition, Life Science Library*. New York: Time Life Books, 1967.

Shelton, Herbert M., *Superior Nutrition*. San Antonio, Texas: Willow Publishing, Inc., 1994.

Sherwood, Lauralee, *Human Physiology, From Cells to Systems*. Belmont, California: Wadsworth Publishing Company, 1997.